NATURALLY

NATURALLY

Your Journey to Good Health

Dr Cijith Sreedhar, BNYS

Popular Prakashan
www.popularprakashan.com
authors UPFRONT

Published by Popular Prakashan Private Limited and
AuthorsUpFront Publishing Services Private Limited
info@popularprakashan.com

First Published in 2025

Dr Cijith Sreedhar asserts the moral right to be identified as the author of this work.

ISBN: 978-81-993948-4-1

Printed in India by Trinity Academy For Corporate Training Ltd.
Pune

To Dr Lakshmi, my life partner in purpose, and to Bhadra and Devi, whose pure spirits remind me daily of love, grace and divine joy.

Preface
The Bend That Became the Path

"Nothing in life happens by coincidence," wrote Dr Brian Weiss – a line that has always resonated deeply with me, especially when I reflect on my journey to becoming a Naturopathic doctor.

I come from a family with no medical background, no mentors to guide my way and no one to direct me toward a career aligned with my skills or passion. And yet, I found myself walking a path that less than 0.001 percent of people would even consider - to become a Naturopathy & Yoga doctor, a course that at the time almost no one in India had even heard of. Looking back, I realise it was all part of destiny's design.

Medicine was the only professional choice I ever truly considered, not because of parental pressure, but because I genuinely dislike anything to do with numbers. I could never get along with math, and even history dates felt like a burden. But the human body? That fascinated me. It was in secondary school that this fascination was truly ignited thanks to Miss Jayanthi, my Biology teacher. Through her love for the subject and her ability to make the complex simple, she turned an average student into one of her best.

So after 10th grade I naturally chose Biology to avoid Mathematics. But Physics still haunted me. Though I performed reasonably well, my medical entrance exam scores weren't enough to secure a seat in Modern Medicine, thanks to the fact that 40 percent of the questions came from physics. I still remember reading questions like: "A car moves to the right at 60 km/h and another to the left at 40 km/h. What is the height of the post in the middle?", and feeling utterly defeated.

Being from Kerala, a land with a deep Ayurvedic legacy, my natural fall back was to consider Ayurveda. The first turning point in my life came when my uncle, Prasana Kumar, mentioned his acquaintance with the prominent spiritual and educational group JSS Mahavidyapeetha, Mysore. With his reference, my father went to Mysore to secure a seat for me in their Ayurveda college. But during a casual conversation there, someone mentioned that they also had a college in Ooty offering a course in Naturopathy & Yoga. That evening, my father shared this update casually over the phone.

At that time I wasn't particularly fascinated by Naturopathy. Honestly, I didn't even know what it truly meant. But I was fascinated by Ooty, South India's most iconic hill station. I quickly chose the course in Ooty not out of passion, but with a little mischievous plan: the BNYS (Bachelor of Naturopathy and Yogic Sciences) course started in October, while the Ayurveda course began in November. I figured I could spend a month enjoying Ooty and then request a transfer, since both colleges were under the same management.

But Ooty has a magic of its own. It holds people close.

And soon, I had more than just one reason to stay.

The first reason: I discovered that BNYS was a full-fledged medical degree. Second: I could escape the struggle of memorising Sanskrit *shlokas*, which would have been a challenge for me in Ayurveda. Despite my parents urging me to switch back, I chose to stay.

Ooty gave me so much more than just a course; it gave me friendships, warmth and moments that would shape me forever. On my very first day in Ooty, I met Dr Anand PG, who would become my classmate, roommate and steadfast friend throughout my entire journey.

Then there was Dr Jincy Sundaran, my junior in college. Over time, she became one of my dearest friends. Her family, who lived close to the college, opened their home and hearts to me. They fed me with warmth, love and delicious food, and gave me a sense of belonging away from home.

Initially, my college life was more about friendships and fun than academics. But that changed when I met Sri Krishnappa *ji*, a veteran RSS leader and cancer survivor, during a camp. When I told him I was studying Naturopathy, his eyes lit up with genuine joy and compassion.

"Oh! A Naturopathy student? You can do miracles," he said, with love and conviction.

I was surprised. But when he shared his story, I was moved. Diagnosed with cancer in his 50s, he had refused conventional treatment after being told he'd live only five more years – and that too, bedridden. He chose natural healing instead. Thirty years later, he was still active, travelling and living with purpose. That conversation became a turning point. I realised I wasn't there by accident; I had been chosen. This was the right path.

But that was just the beginning. Destiny had more plans to shape me into a healer.

During my internship, I had one of the most cherished encounters of my life: I met Dr Babu Joseph, the then Director of the National Institute of Naturopathy, Pune. A man of quiet strength and profound wisdom, he would leave a lifelong imprint on me. In Pune, I still carried the habit – the need – to read the Malayalam newspaper every day. But due to financial constraints, I couldn't afford to buy it. Someone told me that the institute library had one, but it belonged to the Director himself.

Driven by desperation (and maybe a bit of stupidity), I walked straight into his cabin and asked, "Sir, can I get the Malayalam newspaper?"

He looked at me, face unreadable, and asked sternly, "For what? To read, or to take with you?"

I replied, with a touch of arrogance that only an idiot could justify. "If it's your personal copy, I'll just read it here. But if it belongs to the institute, I'd prefer to take it with me."

He looked at me, his voice firmer this time: "It's mine, but you can read it. Just leave it here."

His words were strict, but behind them was silent kindness, a subtle permission. That was our first interaction. Little did I know that it would mark the beginning of something extraordinary. Dr Babu Joseph didn't just share his newspaper, he shared his vast knowledge, deep compassion and the humility of a true healer. His presence taught me more than any medical textbook ever could.

After my internship, I had the privilege to work under him at his hospital in Kerala, as a resident medical officer. And it was there that I met the love of my life, Dr Lakshmi. Being from the same field, our journey in true healing has been one of shared vision, values and growth.

Later, another beautiful phase unfolded when I became a visiting consultant at the Amrita School of Ayurveda, under the divine guidance of Mata Amritanandamayi Devi. My role there was to teach basics of Naturopathy & Yoga to Ayurveda students, but I ended up learning much more than I taught.

Another magical turn in my life happened when I was introduced to the world of NLP – Neuro-Linguistic Programming – quite accidentally, through a random message I received in a WhatsApp group. My first taste came through Fr Tobi, and the real deep dive began with Muhamad Rafi, aka 'Magical Rafi'. Through this, I was empowered to embrace healing in its most complete sense: the healing of the mind. This added a completely new perspective to my healing attitude. I began to see that in every disease there is always a deeper layer at play – for better or worse – shaped by our values, beliefs and attitudes, which construct the inner world we live by and reflect in our health.

And then came Prakriti Shakti, the Clinic of Natural Medicine by CGH Earth. A serendipitous phone call from Dr Pradeep Damodaran, Secretary of INYGMA, the professional association of Yoga and Naturopathy doctors, informed me about an interview happening in

Kochi, where I was residing at the time. I went, with no real intention to join, only to end up choosing the offer over a government PhD grant I had secured.

At Prakriti Shakti, everything fell into place. I was doing what I loved, where I was meant to be. Working under the visionary Mr Jose Dominic, the legendary figure in the Indian travel sector and a highly respected pioneer of sustainable and responsible tourism, and under the guidance of Mr Siddharth Dominic, CEO of CGH Earth Wellness, redefined my approach to healing. From seeing Naturopathy treatments as a punishment for the 'sins' of living in comfort, I came to understand Naturopathy & Yoga as a doorway to happy healing, health, happiness and wellbeing. I learned to walk with people, not ahead of them, offering compassion, comfort and sustainable transformation. Meeting health seekers from all over the world, travelling, sharing my experiences and spreading the message of self-love and natural healing, each day continues to enrich me.

In this journey from clueless student to who I am now, the people I met, the patients who trusted me, my colleagues who journeyed with me, organisations I worked and volunteered with, and the books I read played a role in shaping me.

Today I live by the humble truth that whatever I know, teach or share does not belong to me. It simply flows through me.

Two sentences have always guided me:

"Everything ends well. If it's not so now, it's not the end; it's just a bend."

"Luck is when opportunity meets preparation."

And so I walk this path, grateful for every bend, every lesson, every patient and every sunrise that reminds me that healing isn't something we do – it's something we allow.

Yours Naturally
Dr Cijith Sreedhar

Acknowledgments

Over the years, a few books and voices have deeply shaped my thinking and expanded my understanding of natural healing. *Textbook of Natural Medicine* by Dr Joseph Pizzorno and Dr Michael Murray provided a scientific foundation for integrative medicine. *Why We Sleep* by Dr Matthew Walker gave me a profound appreciation for the role of rest in healing. *10% Human* by Alanna Collen opened my eyes to the incredible power of the microbiome. *Breath: The New Science of a Lost Art* by James Nestor helped me reconnect with the ancient wisdom of breathwork. *How to Do the Work* by Dr Nicole LePera brought together psychology and self-healing in a powerful, practical way. *Many Lives, Many Masters* by Dr Brian Weiss reminded me of the spiritual dimensions of healing. I've also found tremendous insight in the teachings of Magical Rafi, Director of Magic of Change, Kain Ramsay, the renowned mentor and trainer in Applied Psychology and the Neuroscience-based podcasts by Dr Andrew Huberman, which continue to inform and inspire my practice.

To all the authors, mentors and voices who've guided me along the way, thank you for your wisdom. To every being who has crossed my path, from my family to the patients, colleagues and friends who have shared in this journey, I am deeply grateful. A special thanks to my parents and brothers, in-laws and my beloved wife and daughters for their unwavering support, love and encouragement. Your belief in me has been a constant source of strength.

To the management of CGH Earth group and my colleagues at Prakriti Shakti, thank you for being an integral part of this journey. A special mention to Dr Anand P Gopalakrishnan and Dr Nithila Catherine for taking the time to read the draft and provide invaluable suggestions. Your thoughtful insights have been truly appreciated.

I would like to offer my deepest gratitude to Popular Prakashan and the AuthorsUpFront team who helped bring this book into the world. I am thankful to guidance and unwavering support from Harsha Bhatkal and Manish Purohit. Ramya Sarma, with every careful edit, you gave my words clarity, rhythm, and life. Neena Gupta, your artistry turned a vision into a cover that speaks to the heart and soul of this book. I am profoundly grateful.

Finally, I want to extend my deepest gratitude to you, the reader. Thank you for choosing to spend your time and energy on this book. I recognise the value of your commitment and I believe that within these pages you will find inspiration, knowledge and healing to guide you on your own journey toward well-being. Your willingness to invest in yourself is the first step toward transformation – and for that, I am truly honoured.

Contents

CHAPTER 1

The Perspectives

The Different Perspective of Healing

First of all, let me tell you something important: This is not just about reading a book; it is about embarking on a journey. Not an ordinary journey, but an amazing one that leads to health and healing. A journey that will be exciting, impactful and rewarding.

They say what makes a journey memorable is not just the destination, but the company. In this journey of self-healing, you will have the best companions, the most incredible healing agents, drawn from nature and the innate wisdom of your own body.

Why I Wrote This Book

Let me admit something upfront: I am not someone who enjoys writing. I prefer talking, interacting with people, sharing knowledge and recounting the incredible stories I've encountered as a doctor trained in the extraordinary healing system of Naturopathy & Yoga. For over 15 years I have preached, practiced and proved that the body has an incredible capacity to heal itself, when we give it a chance. Witnessing the amazement on people's faces when they experience this truth excites me to dive deeper into the science of healing. Time and again they have asked me, "How can we connect with this system of healing and refresh ourselves?" So here I am, writing on what I've spoken about countless times: the healer within you.

Let's begin this journey of Self-Healing/ awakening in the healer in you. Get your backpack ready.

Before we kick-start our journey, let's pause to reflect on two key points:

1. Why This Journey Is Important

This journey matters because in today's modern era of information overload, the knowledge of almost anything is just a few clicks away. From the intricate structure of atoms to the complex functioning of rockets that explore the universe, all we need is a smartphone and an internet connection. But here's the real question: How many of us take the time to use this vast resource to truly understand ourselves, our bodies, the cells that form the foundation of our being and the systems that make life possible?

This journey is essential because knowing without doing is no better than not knowing. Even if we are aware, how many of us transform that knowledge into actionable steps to prevent or overcome the greatest suffering of all: ill health and disease?

This journey is important because it will free you from the worst slavery of modern times – dependency on doctors, hospitals and medicines.

This book holds your hand through the journey, guiding you along the path of true healing through Naturopathy & Yoga, a drugless, non-invasive and rational system that harnesses the power of nature. Rooted in the principles of healthy living, this approach restores balance, promotes well-being naturally and empowers you to heal and achieve health by yourself.

Isn't that an exciting journey?

2. This Journey Is for Whom?

The thrilling journey of Naturopathy and Yoga healing is really for those of us who don't want to just follow the crowd. It's for people who are ready to take charge of their own health and make informed choices, rather than letting others decide everything for them. Think about it – how many times do we just accept what we're told, accept the tag of a disease, pop a pill without questioning it? Naturopathy invites us to step away from that, to trust our bodies and take the reins when it comes to our health.

It's also for those who want to stand up for themselves. It's not about passively accepting sickness or disease, but about defending yourself against them with knowledge and empowerment. Naturopathy gives you the tools to be proactive, to understand how your body works and how the right foods and practices can make all the difference.

It's like being in charge of your own healing journey, knowing that you're not just a victim of whatever comes your way, but an active participant in creating your health. You start to realise that sickness doesn't have to be something you simply endure; it can be something you face with strength, with confidence and with the understanding that you have the power to heal.

At its heart, Naturopathy is about empowering you to take control, make informed decisions and live a life where you're not just reacting to health issues, but actively preventing them. You have the tools, and now it's your choice. You get to decide.

Naturopathy healing is for those who know and choose to do, who want to have informed choices in life, who don't want everything to be decided by others, who prefer to stand up for themselves and to defend, who want to get empowered against sickness and disease.

In this journey of health and wellbeing, where do you stand now, and where do you want to go?

Imagine a health scale from 0 to 10:

- 0 represents premature death.
- 10 represents absolute health.

(Premature death refers to life lost due to preventable causes – illnesses or conditions that could have been avoided with timely, effective care. As the

saying goes, "Naturopathy healing is not about dying old, but dying young, as late as possible.")

Pause and reflect: Where would you place yourself on this scale? Let's explore that together.

Understanding Your Position on the Health Scale

If you're between 1 and 4: You may be living with diagnosed diseases or conditions. You might rely on medications to regulate vital signs or lab results. Diseases could be limiting your choices, energy and daily activities. Life often feels like a constant struggle to manage symptoms and prevent decline.

If you're between 7 and 10: You likely enjoy vibrant health, physically, mentally, socially and spiritually. You feel energised, engaged and resilient. Work and life flow with clarity and joy. Even when challenges arise, you meet them with strength and ease.

The Zone of 'False Wellness' (4 to 7)

What if you fall between 4 and 7? This range is tricky – a zone of *false wellness*. Many patients I meet fall here, often saying things like: "I have two stents in my heart, but I'm completely healthy now." Or "I get fevers sometimes, but medicines take care of it."

Sounds familiar? This zone can feel deceptively safe. But in truth, it's a gradual decline unless you act. Without effort, it's easy to slip downward. Climbing upward? That calls for awareness, effort and a conscious decision to break free from your comfort zone.

The Illusion of False Wellness

False wellness is when someone appears outwardly stable but lacks the inner vitality and balance needed for true health. It's marked by:

- Reliance on medications or quick fixes to control symptoms without addressing root causes.

- Acceptance of symptoms as 'normal', ignoring subtle signs of imbalance.
- A belief that the absence of serious illness equals good health, overlooking the potential for vibrant well-being.

Take hypertension, for example. Many patients depend solely on medication to manage blood pressure. These drugs may keep numbers 'normal', but can mask ongoing damage to the heart and blood vessels. Someone might say, "My BP is fine, I'm on medication," but this doesn't reflect real health.

The root cause behind elevated blood pressure is often ignored. Medications artificially control the symptom without solving the underlying issue. Over time, the untreated cause manifests elsewhere as complications or comorbidities.

We're conditioned to accept these as expected outcomes of hypertension or long-term drug use. But in truth, they arise not from the condition itself, but from our failure to address its origin.

Living in this area of false wellness leads us to the trap of the **'Comfort Zone',** managing symptoms with medication while neglecting the body's signals. Over time, complications are accepted as inevitable.

The Comfort Zone and Its Pitfalls

False wellness can feel safe. It demands little and change feels unnecessary. Yet, staying here often results in:

- **Stagnation:** The body and mind stop growing or healing.
- **Complacency:** Issues like pain or dysfunction are ignored until they worsen.
- **Unawareness:** Many don't realise how much better they *could* feel with real healing.

True Health and Spirit: The Transformational Shift

The difference between being in the 4–7 range and achieving the 7–10 range is profound:

- Energy and Vitality: True health brings a sense of lightness and energy that allows you to engage fully with life. False wellness, on the other hand, often leaves you feeling sluggish or burdened.
- Connection to Self: When truly healthy, you feel deeply connected to your body, mind and spirit. You're attuned to your body's needs and can respond to them intuitively.
- Emotional Clarity: True health fosters a sense of emotional balance and mental clarity, while false wellness often includes underlying stress or unresolved emotions.
- Sustainable Wellness: True health is self-sustaining and grows stronger over time. False wellness, however, is fragile and often dependent on external factors like medication or temporary fixes.

My patients express this beautiful, transformative experience as 'I feel connected to my body', 'I feel light and relaxed' or I feel cleansed from my core to my skin'.

The Challenge of Moving Upward

Healing is a process of empowerment, and true empowerment lies beyond your comfort zone. Yes, stepping out of one's comfort zone is challenging. It's like when a train changes tracks – there's often a noticeable jerk. But that shift is absolutely necessary for you to reach your destination.

To move upward on the health scale, you must be willing to:

- Challenge Your Habits: Question what you accept as 'normal' and explore healthier alternatives.
- Invest in Yourself: Commit time, energy and resources to your health journey.

- Embrace Discomfort: Understand that growth often involves temporary discomfort, but leads to lasting transformation.

Reflect and Assess Your Health

Take a moment to truly reflect on your current state of well-being. Be honest with yourself as you note your answer.

The following questions will help you do a self-assessment, rating yourself on a scale of 1 to 10 for each:

1. How well do you adapt to changes in life?
2. How in control do you feel when facing challenges?
3. Are you able to wake up in the morning with excitement for the new day?
4. Can you smile and connect with people around you?
5. How excited and passionate are you about your current profession or social roles?
6. How would you describe your energy levels throughout the day?
7. How often do you feel at peace with yourself and your surroundings?
8. How often can you move your body in ways that feel good to you?
9. Do you make time for self-care and personal growth?
10. How often do you experience a deep sense of gratitude?

Once you've rated yourself, sum up your values and divide the total by 10. This will give you the average score, providing you with a clearer sense of your position on the health scale.

Done? Great! Let's move forward…

Understanding Where You Stand: The First Step Towards Meaningful Change

This honest self-assessment will help you identify areas for growth and improvement. Healing and growth require intention, and the power to move up the health scale is in your hands. It's about more than just achieving 'wellness'; it's about moving towards true vitality.

The journey starts with the choices you make today, and with each step you can make progress toward a more balanced, vibrant life.

If Your Score is Below 7: Embrace Change

From a Naturopathy perspective, *change* is essential to healing. While it's natural to resist, staying stuck in familiar – whether comfortable or chaotic – patterns comes at a cost. To truly heal and grow, we must reflect honestly on our motivations, actions and mindset. Without self-awareness and adaptability, healing stalls, and life can feel unfulfilling.

Change isn't always easy. But in handling these moments with honesty, patience, trust and an open mind, we create space for real healing. In Naturopathy, the best time to begin is always now, because healing is a continuous journey shaped by the choices we make every day.

Embracing the Traits of Healthy Individuals

This way of change enables the development of significant personality traits of 'healthy' individuals. These traits include:

- A deep concern for the well-being of self, others and social causes, extending beyond personal interests.
- The capacity for reflection, transcendence and a profound appreciation of life's simple moments.
- An openness to creativity, originality and the exploration of new ideas and perspectives.
- The ability to form meaningful, fulfilling relationships while also feeling at ease in solitude.
- A strong sense of self-acceptance, free from excessive self-criticism or ego-driven motives.
- Clarity in perceiving reality, with fairness in assessing people and situations.
- Resilience and adaptability in the face of uncertainty, challenge or doubt.

- A mindset focussed on solutions and growth, rather than reaction or blame.
- Spontaneity and playfulness, balanced with thoughtfulness and humour.
- The strength to resist societal pressures without needing to be rebellious or unconventional.

Embracing Change: The First Step Towards True Health

By embracing change and cultivating these qualities, you begin the journey toward becoming a truly healthy, balanced and vibrant individual. The first step is to develop a deeper understanding of health and disease.

Let's continue this journey by exploring the core principles that govern both health and illness, and how you can support your body's natural ability to heal. This is a lifelong path that calls for dedication and commitment, but the rewards of radiant health and a fulfilling life make every step worthwhile.

Step 1: Understanding Health

What is Health?

All of us seek health, want to be healthy and remain healthy. But do we really know what we are looking for? We often hear that health is more than just the absence of disease. But what does that truly mean?

In Naturopathy, health is understood in two essential ways: first, as the body's ability to restore balance on its own; and second, as its ability to adapt and self-manage. It's about how well your body and mind can bounce back from life's challenges.

Health is multidimensional – physical, mental, emotional, social and spiritual. True well-being emerges when these aspects work in harmony, allowing us to heal, adapt and thrive. Think of your health like a garden. A thriving garden isn't free from weeds, storms or pests; it flourishes because it can recover. It adjusts, grows stronger and keeps blooming. Our health works the same way.

Stress, environmental changes and personal struggles will always be part of life. The real question isn't whether challenges arise, but how well we adapt to them. When we're truly healthy, our bodies and minds recover quickly and return to balance, no matter what life throws our way.

Many people assume their well-being depends entirely on external circumstances:

"I'm stressed because my job is demanding."

"I'm not feeling well because the climate is changing."

"I'll be happy again when my relationship is back to normal."

But here's the truth – waiting for life to return to a 'perfect' state isn't the answer. Real health isn't about going back to how things were; it's about finding balance in the now. If you change jobs and feel unsettled, wellness doesn't lie in your old routine; it lies in learning to thrive in the new one.

Resilience isn't just about surviving hard times; it's about growing through them. Picture a tree in a storm. A rigid tree that refuses to bend is more likely to break, while one that sways with the wind survives and continues to grow. Your body and mind are similar. The immune system doesn't only fight infections, it learns and strengthens over time. Your mind too becomes more resilient when you learn to navigate stress rather than simply endure it.

This doesn't mean you should never seek help. Sometimes, we all need guidance, through therapy, medicine or lifestyle changes. But external support should be like a ship's crew guiding the vessel through rough waters, not something you depend on forever. The ultimate goal is to restore your ability to steer your own course.

Health is not a destination; it's an ongoing process of adaptation, growth and healing. Just like a vibrant garden needs regular care to flourish, we need to tend to our health continually. And in the end, true health isn't just about surviving, but about living fully and thriving through all seasons of life.

Looking Beyond Appearances: Metabolic Health

We often associate health with a strong, muscular body. But have you heard of people who looked incredibly fit yet collapsed unexpectedly? That's because having a good physique is just one piece of the puzzle – it doesn't always mean a person is truly healthy.

Your body isn't just muscles. It has 11 major systems, including the heart, liver, kidneys, brain and gut. If one of these isn't functioning well, your overall health suffers, even if your muscles look great. A strong body on the outside doesn't always mean a strong system on the inside. The heart needs to pump efficiently, the liver needs to detoxify, the kidneys need to filter waste and the gut needs to absorb nutrients. When these systems work in harmony, it has what we call 'metabolic health' - you experience real health, with energy, resilience and longevity.

So the next time you think about health, look beyond the mirror. Focus on what's happening inside and be strong, inside and out.

Step 2: Understanding Disease: A Natural Perspective

What is Disease?

Most of us recognise the names of diseases like diabetes, hypertension or arthritis. Yet, when we visit a doctor for the first time, we don't typically say, "I have diabetes" or "I have hypertension" unless we've already self-diagnosed through research. Instead, we approach doctors because we experience discomfort or 'dis-ease'. This disease might manifest in various ways, such as:

- Persistent aches or pains.
- Disturbed sleep or digestion.

- Fatigue or low energy levels.
- Difficulty in memory or communication, or something similar.

Doctors interpret these symptoms, give them a name and often prescribe medication. But does labelling discomfort or taking a pill truly address the problem? The real purpose of seeking medical advice should be to understand why the symptoms occur. When we approach disease with the question "Why?" our entire perception of and response to illness shifts. This mindset helps us see disease as the body's way of communicating an internal imbalance. By viewing symptoms as signals, not enemies, we can better understand the root causes of our discomfort.

Disease as the Body's Communication System

Imagine your body as a finely tuned orchestra, with every organ and cell working in harmony. Disease occurs when something disrupts this balance: a nutritional deficiency, toxin build-up, emotional stress or poor lifestyle habits. These disruptions manifest as disorders in the body's normal functioning.

Symptoms such as pain, fatigue or fever act like a car's warning light, alerting you to underlying issues. For instance:

- Pain: When you sprain your ankle, the pain signals injury and prompts you to rest so that healing can occur.
- Fatigue: Feeling unusually tired could indicate that your body is fighting an infection or coping with stress.
- Fever: This is a natural defence mechanism where your body raises its temperature to eliminate harmful pathogens.

These symptoms are the body's survival mechanisms. They are not the disease itself, but the body's way of restoring balance. Recognising this helps us shift from fearing symptoms to understanding and addressing their cause.

Why Do Symptoms Arise?

Imagine eating stale food. Your body reacts by triggering vomiting to eliminate the harmful substance, a clear sign that it's protecting itself. But if you take medicine to stop the vomiting immediately, you interrupt this defence. Yes, vomiting can sometimes be excessive and require help, but in the early stages, suppressing it may do more harm than good.

The same applies to pain. Taking a painkiller for a headache may ease the discomfort, but it doesn't fix the root cause. Was the pain from dehydration, stress, poor posture or something deeper? Painkillers mute the signal, much like wiping water from a leaking pipe without repairing it – the leak continues, and the damage grows.

Symptoms like pain, fatigue or fever are not random annoyances. They're messages from the body that something is wrong. Suppressing them without understanding why they're there is like 'shooting the messenger'. A headache may be your body's way of warning about stress, eye strain or an internal imbalance. Ignoring the message risks letting the problem worsen.

Picture a king at war who receives troubling reports from the battlefield. If he kills the messengers to avoid bad news, he's not solving the problem; he's avoiding reality. The true issue lies on the battlefield, not with the messengers. Similarly, symptoms are messengers alerting us to an inner struggle between health and disease. Silencing them doesn't stop the conflict; it just delays action.

Our bodies are always balancing healing forces against those that cause illness. When symptoms appear, they signal where support is needed. Suppressing these signs means we miss the chance to help the body restore harmony.

Addressing the root cause – drinking water for dehydration, resting for fatigue or managing stress – supports the body's healing capacity.

When we respond to the message rather than ignore it, we shift toward real recovery instead of a temporary fix.

Just as it's unwise for a king to silence messengers, it's unwise for us to suppress symptoms without understanding their cause. Instead, by decoding and responding to them, we support healing and move closer to lasting health, not just the illusion of it.

Diseases as Broken Biochemistry: A Naturopathic Perspective

In Naturopathy, one foundational concept is that diseases stem from disruptions or imbalances in the body's biochemistry. This perspective views illness not merely as isolated symptoms, but as the result of broken or malfunctioning cellular processes. Biochemistry, the intricate web of chemical reactions that sustains life, is at the core of this understanding. When these processes are disrupted, the result is a cascade of dysfunction that manifests as disease. By addressing these underlying biochemical imbalances, Naturopathy aims to restore harmony and support the body's innate ability to heal.

Biochemistry: Understanding the Chemical Basis of Life and Disease

I have to explain some complicated stuff here, but it is important. Biochemistry is the branch of science that studies the chemical processes and substances that occur within living organisms. It focusses on the molecular level, examining how molecules like proteins, lipids, carbohydrates and other nutrients interact and contribute to cellular function, growth, reproduction and repair. At its core, Biochemistry is about how the body converts raw materials (food, water and oxygen) into energy, builds and repairs structures, and regulates processes to maintain life. These processes are tightly controlled and rely on precise interactions between molecules.

Understanding Biochemistry in Cells

Our body is made up of tiny cells; inside those cells there are many processes happening all the time to keep us healthy. Biochemistry is like the 'recipe book' of the cell, explaining how everything works together. Here are the main parts:

1. Enzymes: Think of enzymes as helpers that speed up important processes in the body. They make biochemical reactions happen faster, helping the body get what it needs.
2. Metabolic Pathways: These are like highways inside your cells. They help turn food into energy (like ATP), build things your body needs and get rid of waste, making sure that all is well inside you.
3. Molecular Signals: Our body needs a way to communicate with its different parts. Molecules like hormones and neurotransmitters help cells talk to each other and keep everything running smoothly.
4. Genetic Regulation: DNA is like an instruction manual for making the proteins that do most of the work in the body. RNA helps 'read' the instructions and make sure things happen as they should.

When biochemistry is working well, our cells do their jobs properly, and we stay healthy. But if something goes wrong, it can cause problems in the body.

What Can Go Wrong in Biochemistry?

Several things can mess up how our cells work. Here's how:

1. Nutritional Deficiencies: Our cells need certain vitamins, minerals and other nutrients to work properly. Without them, things get stuck. For example:
    - If you're low in Vitamin D, your bones can weaken.
    - If you're low in iron, it can make you feel tired and anaemic.
2. Inflammation: Sometimes the body gets too worked up and starts attacking itself, causing pain and damage. Chronic inflammation can lead to conditions like arthritis, diabetes and heart disease. (refer: Box - Inflammation: The Paradoxical Fire)

3. Genetic Mutations and Errors: Our genes are like the body's instruction manual. If there's a mistake in the instructions (like a genetic mutation), it can cause problems. For example, if the instructions for repairing cellular damage are messed up, it can lead to cancer.
4. Toxin Exposure: Harmful substances in the environment, like pollution or chemicals, can disrupt the body's processes.
5. For instance: Lead can hurt the brain, making it harder to think clearly. Drinking alcohol can damage the liver, making it harder to process fats.
6. Hormonal Imbalances: Hormones are like messages that tell the body what to do. If there's too much or too little of certain hormones, things can go wrong, resulting conditions like thyroid disorders.

Step 3: Disorders: The Underlying Causes of Diseases

Diseases that manifest as symptoms arise due to underlying disorders in the body. It is crucial to understand that no disease exists without an underlying disorder, even if the exact disorder is sometimes difficult to detect.

As doctors, we may be able to pinpoint the precise disorder in some cases, while in others it might remain undetected due to the complexities of human physiology or limitations of diagnostic tools. However, every disease has a root cause, which is a disorder.

These underlying disorders can be broadly classified into five major categories:

- Developmental Disorders
- Metabolic Disorders
- Degenerative Disorders
- Neoplastic Disorders
- Pathogenic Disorders

Inflammation: The Paradoxical Fire

Inflammation: The word *inflammation* hints at its nature – it means to 'inflame', like a fire burning inside. Like fire, inflammation can be helpful when controlled, providing warmth, defence and healing. But if it rages unchecked, it causes destruction. Inflammation works the same way: vital for healing, yet harmful if persistent.

The Two Sides of Inflammation

Acute Inflammation: The Body's First Responder

Acute inflammation is the body's fast response to injury or infection, like an emergency team at a crisis location. The immune system detects a problem – such as a cut or invading bacteria – and sends white blood cells to resolve it. This short-term response is essential for healing.

Classic Signs of Acute Inflammation

1. **Redness** – Increased blood flow delivers immune cells.
2. **Swelling** – Fluid and immune cells accumulate to fight threats.
3. **Heat** – A slight rise in temperature helps kill microbes.
4. **Pain** – Signals the body to rest and protect the area.

Once healing begins, the inflammation fades and balance is restored.

Chronic Inflammation: The Hidden Danger

Chronic inflammation is like a fire that smoulders without a clear cause. Instead of healing, it causes slow, ongoing damage. Unlike acute inflammation, which is obvious and short-lived, chronic inflammation is silent and long-term, often going unnoticed until serious harm is done.

Inflammation: The Paradoxical Fire (*contd.*)

Why Chronic Inflammation is Hard to Detect

Imagine a company where an employee steals a large sum; the management reacts swiftly, like acute inflammation. But what if the theft is small and steady over years? It may be missed until the company collapses. That's chronic inflammation, subtle but dangerous over time.

Diseases Linked to Chronic Inflammation

Chronic inflammation plays a key role in many serious conditions:

- **Heart Disease** – Damages vessels, leading to plaque build-up and heart attacks.
- **Diabetes** – Inflammatory chemicals interfere with insulin.
- **Cancer** – Creates conditions where damaged cells grow uncontrollably.
- **Arthritis** – Inflammation in joints causes pain and stiffness.
- **Autoimmune Diseases** – The immune system attacks healthy tissues.
- **Alzheimer's Disease** – Brain inflammation contributes to memory loss.
- **Asthma and Allergies** – Persistent airway inflammation leads to breathing issues.

Understanding inflammation is vital. Acute inflammation defends and heals, but chronic inflammation becomes a hidden threat. Recognising its signs helps us take action, supporting long-term health and resilience.

Though each category has defining characteristics, it is also important to note that disorders often overlap, meaning that a single disease can have characteristics of multiple categories.

1. Developmental Disorders (Genetic Disorders)

Developmental disorders are conditions that affect how tissues and organs grow, develop or take shape. These issues often start before birth, but some might only show up later in life. They usually happen due to something going wrong during foetal development or early childhood.

Genes – that are made up of DNA – tell your body how to grow, develop and function. They guide the production of proteins, which are the building blocks that help your body do everything from forming tissues to managing chemical reactions.

You inherit your genes from both parents, and they influence things like your eye colour, hair type and how your organs form and work. But sometimes these genes can have mutations, or small changes that don't follow the usual plan. These changes can come from your parents or be triggered by things like infections, toxins or other environmental factors during pregnancy.

When this happens, it can lead to developmental disorders that affect your body physically, mentally or functionally. For example, a gene mutation related to heart development could cause a congenital heart defect. If a gene that guides brain growth is affected, it might lead to challenges with learning, behaviour or mental skills.

Some of these issues are obvious at birth, like certain physical abnormalities, while others like cognitive or behavioural challenges might not become clear until later. Either way, these conditions are rooted in how our genes guide development, and when something goes off track, the effects can vary widely.

2. Metabolic Disorders

Metabolism refers to the essential chemical reactions that convert the food we eat into energy, support tissue growth and repair, and manage waste elimination. These processes depend on enzymes, hormones and various bodily systems working in harmony.

Metabolic disorders occur when these chemical processes are disrupted, whether in how the body produces energy, breaks down nutrients or eliminates waste. While these disorders can affect the entire body, they often impact key organs like the liver, pancreas or kidneys, which play central roles in metabolism.

The diseases commonly known as lifestyle diseases are, at their core, metabolic disorders. The term **metabolic syndrome** describes a cluster of conditions arising from underlying metabolic imbalances. These typically include elevated blood pressure, high blood sugar, excess abdominal fat and abnormal cholesterol or triglyceride levels.

3. Degenerative Disorders

Degenerative disorders involve the slow and steady breakdown of tissues, cells or organs over time. To really understand how this happens, it helps to first look at how the body naturally repairs itself. The human body has an amazing built-in system for renewal. Cells in tissues like skin, blood and bone are constantly being replaced. For instance, skin cells renew every few weeks, while bones continuously rebuild to stay strong. This ongoing repair is powered by stem cells, growth factors and enzymes that fix damaged tissues.

But degeneration begins when this repair system can't keep up with the damage. This imbalance might be caused by ageing, long-term stress on tissues, poor nutrition, environmental toxins or even genetics. Over time, the damage starts to outweigh the body's ability to fix itself, leading to gradual and often permanent breakdown. A good example is osteoarthritis, where the cartilage in joints wears down from repeated use and limited repair, causing pain and stiffness.

Although we usually associate these disorders with old age, younger people can be affected too, especially if their bodies are exposed to long-term stress, unhealthy habits or inherited risks.

4. Neoplastic Disorders

While growth and division are essential functions of most body cells, their uncontrolled and abnormal activity can result in tumour formation, referred to as neoplasms. These tumours can be benign (non-cancerous) or malignant (cancerous). Unlike disorders involving cell destruction, neoplasms result from unchecked cell creation. Since growth is usually seen as a positive process, the body often fails to detect it as a threat. As a result, many neoplastic growths remain asymptomatic for a long time. With no signal to halt the process, the body doesn't initiate repair or defence mechanisms.

Benign tumours grow slowly and stay localised. They don't invade surrounding tissues or spread to other parts of the body. Still, they can cause problems if they press against vital structures. A benign brain tumour might trigger headaches or vision problems by compressing nearby areas.

Malignant tumours, commonly referred to as cancer, grow aggressively, invade nearby tissues and may spread to distant organs through the blood or lymphatic system in a process known as metastasis. Their ability to affect multiple body systems makes them more dangerous and harder to treat.

Usually, cells grow, divide and die in an orderly manner. However, when this natural cycle is disrupted, cells may begin to multiply uncontrollably. This loss of control is often driven by gene mutations caused by toxins, radiation, viruses or inherited traits that interfere with the normal regulation of cell growth, leading to neoplastic development.

Mental and emotional health also play a surprisingly big role in how the body handles abnormal cell growth. Recent research shows that chronic stress, unresolved trauma and long-term anxiety can weaken the immune system and interfere with the body's ability to regulate cells properly. These emotional challenges don't just affect how we feel, but can actually act as triggers or contributing factors in the development of cancer. More studies are confirming what many traditional healing systems have long believed: the mind-body connection is real and incredibly powerful.

Examples of neoplastic disorders include **breast cancer**, a common malignant tumour that can spread to other parts of the body if not detected early; **lipoma**, a benign fatty tumour that typically forms under the skin and may cause discomfort if it grows large; and **leukaemia**, a cancer of the blood-forming tissues where abnormal white blood cells multiply uncontrollably, crowding out healthy cells and impairing the immune system.

5. Pathogenic Disorders (Infections)

Pathogenic disorders are different from other types of disorders because they are communicable, meaning that they can spread from one person to another. These disorders are caused by infections from harmful organisms known as pathogens, which include bacteria, viruses, fungi or parasites. When these pathogens enter the body, they can disrupt normal body functions and cause a variety of health problems.

Pathogenic infections can be either acute (short-term) or chronic (long-term), and in some cases may lead to more serious complications such as sepsis, which is a life-threatening response to infection. Certain infections can also trigger other health issues, such as autoimmune or inflammatory disorders, where the body mistakenly attacks its own tissues.

Overlapping Disorders - Manifestation as Diseases

Disorders often do not manifest as diseases in a straightforward way; instead, they are interlinked and overlap with one another. This means that one condition can lead to or exacerbate another, creating a complex web of health issues. Many diseases are multifactorial, meaning they arise from a combination of factors from different categories of disorders, such as metabolic, pathogenic or genetic issues. For example, someone with a metabolic disorder like Type 2 diabetes may develop additional complications like neuropathy or retinopathy, due to the impact of the disease on the body. Similarly, a pathogenic disorder like HIV/AIDS not only weakens the immune system, but can also lead to degenerative changes in the body.

Cancer may arise from a genetic predisposition, but its manifestation and severity are often influenced by metabolic factors. Understanding how these factors overlap is crucial for adopting a more holistic approach to diagnosis and management. It shifts our focus from merely managing symptoms to addressing the root causes. Most diseases begin with an underlying imbalance in the body, which disrupts normal function and eventually leads to illness. By identifying and correcting these imbalances, we support the body's natural ability to heal and maintain health.

Step 4: Understanding Imbalances - The Root Cause of Diseases

So far, we've explored how diseases are forms of communication from within, and behind every disease there's a disorder. But what initiates these messages? They don't arise from nowhere; there's always a reason. That reason lies in the imbalances within our cells. When we experience imbalances, the body responds with disease. Put positively, when we maintain balance the body maintains health. Health and disease are simply responses of the body to how we treat it.

Our health and diseases are deeply tied to the internal balance of our bodies. Rather than viewing disease as caused by a single factor, it helps to understand the body as a complex, interconnected system. Imbalance isn't only about physical or chemical issues; it also includes deeper misalignments within our body, mind and spirit. These can manifest in different ways, and by recognising them we gain more power over our health and healing.

In traditional healing systems like Chinese medicine and Ayurveda, disease is seen as a result of imbalance, be it between Yin and Yang or among the three *doshas*. But for most people, these ideas may feel abstract. Naturopathy makes it simpler. Instead of complex theories, it teaches that when we stray from our natural state due to ignorance, stress, fear, greed, cravings or societal pressure, we create inner conflict, and illness follows. In other words, when we're out of sync with our body's true needs, imbalance arises and disease sets in.

Many of these imbalances begin at the cellular level. Our body is made up of trillions of cells, each with vital tasks. When these cells are out of balance, they struggle to function, affecting tissues, organs and ultimately, our overall health. These cellular imbalances, shaped by both internal and external factors, create a ripple effect that touches everything from energy and immunity to genetic expression.

So, most health issues are the result of multiple imbalances that lead to disorders and eventually, disease. By understanding and addressing these imbalances, we begin to heal more deeply. In the next section, we'll explore the types of imbalances that can disrupt the harmony of body and mind and how they contribute to disease. If we can correct them, the body can return to health. Let's explore this further.

What Imbalances Are Present in Your Body?

Imagine your body as a well-organised, bustling city. When all systems in the city function harmoniously, life thrives. But when imbalances occur, it's like parts of the city breaking down, leading to chaos and eventually disease. These imbalances fall into several key categories:

1. Assimilative Imbalance: Fuelling Your Body's Engine

Think of your body like a car. To run smoothly, it needs quality fuel and all its parts working in harmony. The essential raw materials your body needs are simple: food, water, air and sunlight. These are the basic ingredients it uses to stay healthy and function properly. But it's not just about giving your body these inputs - it also needs the right conditions to make use of them.

This is where assimilation plays a key role. Assimilation is the process of taking in these raw materials and using them to keep the body running well. For instance, when you eat, your body needs to digest food and absorb its nutrients. If it doesn't get enough or the right kind of nutrients, things can go off track. You might feel sluggish, experience indigestion or suffer from fatigue. It's like trying to run a car on poor-quality fuel - it simply won't perform well.

But giving your body the right input isn't enough. It also needs time and space to use them efficiently. This includes getting enough sleep, staying active and allowing time to relax and de-stress. During rest, exercise and sleep, your body uses nutrients to repair cells, restore energy and keep systems running smoothly.

What happens if you don't give your body these chances? Without enough sleep, movement or relaxation, it can't make full use of the good fuel you provide. You might feel drained, your immune system could weaken or your digestion might slow, making it harder to absorb nutrients.

2. Defence and Repair Imbalances: The Body's Army

The defence and repair in our body is handled by the immune system, which acts like a nation's army – constantly alert and ready to protect us from external threats like pathogens. Imagine a king with a powerful army who neglects its upkeep. Instead of strengthening his own forces, he hires outsiders to fight for him. Sometimes they win, sometimes they don't, but each time the king loses a bit of his land. Is that a wise strategy? Clearly not.

Now apply this to our bodies. We have a capable immune system, yet we often fail to support it properly. The immune system protects against harmful invaders like bacteria, viruses and fungi. It also keeps watch for damaged or abnormal cells, such as cancer cells, and eliminates them early. During injuries or infections, it promotes tissue repair and healing. It regulates inflammation so that it doesn't spiral out of control, as chronic inflammation. It even has a memory, enabling quicker responses to known threats. Most importantly, it maintains balance, strong enough to fight infections, yet smart enough not to attack healthy cells. It's like a skilled security force constantly guarding our health.

Like any army, the immune system needs both skill and discipline. Without skill, it leaves us vulnerable to infection. Without discipline, it may attack the body itself, leading to autoimmune disorders. Neither is ideal. What we truly need is a balanced immune system.

To keep it effective, we must help it stay both strong and well-regulated. This involves managing immune responses, controlling inflammation and handling infections efficiently. Think of it as maintaining a powerful yet dependable army – ready to protect, but never overreacting.

Yet, instead of supporting this powerful system with healthy habits, we often turn to quick fixes like pills. While they may offer short-term relief, they can also bring side effects that weaken the immune system over time, leading to chronic issues like autoimmune disorders on one end of the health scale and frequent infections on the other.

3. Energy Imbalances: Powering the City

Energy drives every function in your body, much like electricity powers a city. The source, timing and quality of this energy play a vital role in maintaining balance. Inside your cells, tiny structures called mitochondria produce energy. You may recall from school biology that mitochondria are the 'powerhouse of the cell'. They act like a car engine, converting fuel into usable energy. But just like an engine, poor-quality fuel or malfunctioning parts can lead to more toxins than energy. One such by-product is free radicals.

Free radicals are toxic substances naturally created during energy production. Think of them as sparks from a misfiring engine. When everything functions well, the body cleans up these sparks efficiently.

But when mitochondria don't work properly, they generate too many free radicals. These unstable molecules move freely through the body, damaging cells, proteins and DNA. Over time, this leads to inflammation, chronic conditions and diseases like diabetes, heart issues and accelerated ageing.

The energy system in your body depends on two main things: the quality of the fuel (nutrient-rich, whole foods) and the efficiency of the mitochondria. Equally important is the timing of energy use. Ideally, you should feel energetic during the day and relaxed by evening to allow restful sleep. However, many people experience the opposite, feeling wired at night and sluggish during the day, disrupting their sleep and daily performance.

When energy production is off-balance, it creates problems. Too little energy during the day causes fatigue, sluggishness and even depression. Excess energy at the wrong time may show up as anxiety, restlessness or feeling constantly 'on edge'.

4. Biotransformation and Elimination: How Your Body Clears Out the Garbage

Think of your body like a busy city that constantly produces waste. To keep things running smoothly, a team of hardworking organs – the liver, kidneys, intestines, lungs and skin – work together to process and remove harmful substances. These toxins come from two main sources. First, external toxins like chemicals, pesticides, pollution and harmful compounds in food, such as charred meat. Second, internal toxins, which are natural by-products of processes like digestion, metabolism or immune responses.

When your detox systems are functioning well, your body clears waste efficiently. But if they get overwhelmed – especially from a build-up of external toxins – trouble starts. Toxins can accumulate, causing inflammation, cellular stress and chronic health problems over time. That's why staying hydrated, eating clean and occasionally doing a gentle detox can help your body's 'waste management' stay efficient.

In Naturopathy, this build-up is known as toxaemia and is seen as the root cause of all disease. This idea is called the Unity of Disease, where an overload of toxins disrupts the body's systems and leads to dysfunction. As eliminative organs get stressed and start to fail, the result is inflammation and chronic illness, particularly in organs involved in detoxification, like the liver, kidneys and skin.

Naturopathy also offers a solution: the Unity of Cure, which focusses on eliminating toxins to restore health. By clearing toxic overload, the body's balance and healing mechanisms can return. That's why supporting your eliminative organs is essential.

While our bodies are designed to manage internal toxins well, today's external toxic load is heavier than ever. It's like a police force meant to handle local issues being overwhelmed by constant attacks from the outside. As attention shifts to external threats, internal waste piles up, worsening the burden.

By addressing toxaemia through detoxification and supporting your body's natural healing, you can protect your health, prevent chronic disease and keep your system working at its best.

5. Communication Imbalances: The Body's Messaging System

For anything to work smoothly – whether it's a company, a family or a team – good communication is essential. The same is true for our body, which is one of the most complex systems you can imagine. It has its own messaging network made up of blood circulation, nerves, hormones, enzymes and brain chemicals called neurotransmitters. These messengers help different parts of the body talk to each other, ensuring that everything works in sync, allowing all the cells and organs to work together like a well-coordinated orchestra.

Each part of this network has a unique role:

- The nervous system is like the body's control room, sending lightning-fast messages between the brain and the rest of the body.

- The endocrine system uses hormones as messengers to regulate things like metabolism, growth and mood. These messages are slower but long-lasting.
- The circulatory system acts as the delivery service, carrying oxygen, nutrients and hormones to cells, and removing waste.
- The immune system communicates threats like infections, helping the body respond and maintain internal order.
- Neurotransmitters act as the body's chemical messengers, enabling communication between nerve cells and influencing mood, memory and behaviour.
- Holistic views also consider energy pathways like meridians and *chakras*, which are believed to influence overall well-being.

When this communication system is running well, your body feels balanced and healthy. But when there's a miscommunication or breakdown, things can go wrong. For example:

- In neuropathy, often linked to diabetes or nerve injuries, damaged nerves can't send signals to and from the brain, leading to numbness, tingling or weakness.
- In mental health issues, brain chemicals like serotonin or dopamine may be out of balance, leading to conditions like depression or anxiety.

When your body's messaging system is clear and effective, everything works as it should, helping you feel healthier and more in tune with your body.

6. Structural Integrity Imbalances: The Body's Foundation

The structural integrity of the body refers to the optimal alignment, function and strength of its systems, ensuring overall health and balance. At its core, this means how well your body parts are aligned, working together, and staying resilient. When everything functions in harmony, the body feels balanced and strong. The musculoskeletal system – bones, muscles, ligaments, tendons and fascia – forms the foundation. These elements support movement, maintain posture and protect against injury. Like a well-built house with a solid frame, a stable musculoskeletal system keeps the body sturdy. Good posture, flexible joints and coordinated movements help maintain this balance.

Structural integrity also includes the protective barriers within the body. Blood vessels have an inner lining called the endothelium that ensures smooth blood flow, prevents leakage and regulates exchange. The gut lining absorbs nutrients, supports immunity and blocks harmful substances. It also helps balance the gut microbiome – the trillions of microbes essential for digestion and overall health. The brain is protected by the blood-brain barrier, a filter that blocks toxins while allowing nutrients to enter. Even deeper, the body depends on genetic integrity – well-maintained DNA that allows cells to repair, function properly and avoid disease.

When these systems are disrupted, structural integrity begins to fail. Poor posture, injuries, inactivity or repetitive motions can misalign the musculoskeletal system, leading to weak joints or muscle imbalances. The endothelial lining may be harmed by inflammation, oxidative stress or high blood pressure, increasing vascular risks. The gut lining can be damaged by stress, poor diet, infections or overuse of antibiotics and painkillers, causing conditions like ulcers or leaky gut. The blood-brain barrier weakens with chronic inflammation or toxin exposure, raising the risk of neurological issues. And DNA damage – whether from toxins, poor nutrition or radiation – can impair cellular repair and lead to serious diseases.

When structural integrity breaks down, it can set off a cascade of problems. Misalignment may lead to scoliosis, disc issues or tendinitis. Damaged blood vessels can result in hypertension or arterial blockages. A compromised gut lining may trigger conditions like IBS, IBD or leaky gut syndrome. Weakness in the blood-brain barrier has been

> **Mitochondria – The Powerhouse of the Cell**
>
> Mitochondria are tiny structures inside our cells that act like power plants. They take the food we eat and turn it into energy that our body can use. This energy, called ATP (adenosine triphosphate), powers everything we do – walking, thinking, even breathing.
>
> Mitochondria also helps in other important functions like cell growth, healing and protecting against damage. They have their own DNA, which means they can partly control how they function. When mitochondria don't work well, it can lead to tiredness and various health problems. Keeping them healthy through good food, exercise and proper rest helps our body stay strong and energetic.

linked to Alzheimer's, Parkinson's and multiple sclerosis. Accumulated DNA damage may contribute to cancer and inherited diseases.

The Connection between Imbalances and Disorders

The human body is an intricate system where everything is deeply interconnected. Health issues rarely stem from a single imbalance; instead, they are often the result of multiple factors working together. An imbalance in the immune system can lead to inflammation. This inflammation doesn't stop there; it can manifest as hundreds of different diseases. Many inflammatory conditions, like arthritis (inflammation of the joints), gastritis (inflammation of the stomach lining) or colitis (inflammation of the colon) are examples of how a single imbalance can create a wide range of disorders.

What makes this even more complex is that the imbalance behind a disease is rarely simple. Instead, it's a combination of several interconnected problems. For instance, diabetes might result from poor nutrition, chronic stress, immune system dysfunction, faulty insulin signalling and even genetic predisposition. The same root imbalances might lead to very different diseases in different people, such as arthritis in one person or cardiovascular disease in another. This multifaceted relationship shows how imbalances can ripple through the body, affecting various systems in unique ways.

Moving Toward True Healing

Naturopathy recognises this complexity and focusses on a holistic approach to health. Instead of treating just the symptoms of a disorder, it aims to identify and address the root causes of the imbalance. This is based on the understanding that the body has an innate ability to heal itself when supported correctly.

A holistic approach in naturopathy considers the whole person, body, mind and environment. Treating diabetes involves more than just managing blood sugar levels. It might include improving nutrition, reducing stress, removing fear and insecurities, supporting immune function and correcting metabolic imbalances. By addressing these interconnected factors, naturopathy helps restore balance, preventing complications and promoting long-term health.

True healing in naturopathy is about creating an environment where the body can thrive. This means focussing on natural therapies, lifestyle changes and personalised care to support the body's ability to heal itself. By looking at the big picture and understanding the deep connections between imbalances and disorders, naturopathy provides a path to health that is both comprehensive and sustainable.

CHAPTER 2

The Healer

The Healing Power of the Body: A Conversation about Nature, Balance and Medicine

The Role of Naturopathy in Healing

The core belief in naturopathy is that the body has an incredible ability to heal itself, as long as it's given the right conditions.

Does the Body Heal Itself?

Have you ever been amazed at how your body seems to take care of itself? When you get a fever, it rises to fight off infection. When you cut yourself, the skin starts to repair and the wound begins to heal. Even when a part of your body is damaged, like when you lose a portion of your liver, it has the ability to regenerate – up to two-thirds of it can grow back to its normal size. All of this happens without you consciously thinking about it. Your body is constantly working behind the scenes to restore balance and bring itself back to a healthy state.

It's nothing short of remarkable how the body heals itself, and this ability is a cornerstone of Naturopathy, an approach to health that emphasises natural healing and the body's innate capacity to repair itself.

The Body's Natural Healing Mechanisms

To understand why the body heals itself, it helps to know a bit about how this process actually works. The body has an innate intelligence, an internal wisdom that quietly manages everything from repairing tissues to fighting infections and maintaining balance.

Take a simple cut, for example. Your body jumps into action right away. Blood vessels narrow to slow bleeding, platelets form a clot and white blood cells rush in to fight off bacteria. Then, new skin starts to grow, eventually closing the wound and forming a scar. You don't have to think about it, it just happens.

The same goes for something more serious, like a broken bone. As soon as the break occurs, the body begins repairing it. Special cells form new bone tissue, gradually fusing the bone back together. A cast or surgery might support this process, but the real healing comes from within. Without the body's own repair systems, those medical tools wouldn't be nearly as effective.

This ability to restore and maintain balance is part of what's known as homeostasis. Whether it's healing an injury, fighting off germs or keeping body temperature steady, your body is always working to stay balanced. And when it's in balance, healing happens more efficiently.

That's the beauty of the body; it's built to heal. But it needs the right support. Naturopathy focuses on creating the conditions that let your body do what it's naturally designed to do: heal and thrive. It's not about fixing you from the outside, but about helping your body do its job better from the inside.

Understanding how your body heals – and what gets in the way – gives you the power to take charge of your health.

Naturopathy is about:

1. Supporting the Body's Natural Healing Capacity: It addresses the root causes of imbalance, helping your body restore itself to a normal, functional state.
2. Promoting Adaptability: True health includes the ability to adapt to environmental, physical and emotional stressors. Naturopathy helps you build resilience, enabling your body to recover from challenges without relying on external interventions.
3. Holistic Wellness: Healing is about the whole being – physical, emotional, mental and spiritual. Naturopathy helps restore balance in all of these areas for lasting well-being.

4. Prevention and Longevity: By focussing on lifestyle practices, diet and natural remedies, naturopathy promotes long-term vitality and helps prevent illness before it starts.

Through this concepts and approach, naturopathy aims to create not just a healthy body but a thriving individual.

Why Naturopathy & Yoga?

In India, Naturopathy & Yoga are combined as a single medical system, often referred to as the two wheels of a cart. They complement each other seamlessly, both being drugless healing modalities that align in philosophy and approach. Doctors qualified to practice Naturopathy & Yoga are awarded the medical degree BNYS (Bachelor of Naturopathy and Yogic Sciences), a five-and-a-half-year medical course, with opportunities for higher studies such as an MD in the field.

Throughout this book and this journey of healing, I will frequently refer to Yoga. Before proceeding further, let me provide a brief explanation of Yoga and its significance.

Yoga: A Path for Liberation, A Tool for Health and Healing

Yoga is one of India's greatest contributions to humanity, offering a path to inner peace and self-realisation. Originally, it was developed to attain *moksha* – liberation from the cycle of birth and rebirth, which is considered the ultimate goal of life in Indian philosophy.

Think of a mug filled with seawater. Though it holds the same essence as the vast ocean, it's limited by the container. Likewise, our soul is divine but confined within the body. As the body ages and eventually dies, the soul doesn't always merge back into the supreme consciousness. Often, it enters another body, continuing the cycle of suffering and attachment. Yoga is developed as a tool to break this cycle, helping us reconnect with our true, divine essence.

There are four main paths in Yoga, each guiding us toward liberation. *Jnana Yoga* is the path of knowledge, where one realises that the material world is impermanent and only the supreme soul is real. *Bhakti Yoga* is the path of devotion, encouraging surrender to the divine and freedom from attachment. *Karma Yoga* focuses on selfless action – doing one's duty without expecting results. *Raja Yoga*, the 'royal path', offers a structured approach involving ethics, breath control, meditation and deep spiritual absorption.

Raja Yoga, as compiled by the sage Patanjali, describes an eightfold path known as *Ashtanga Yoga*. It includes physical postures (*asanas*), breath regulation (*pranayama*) and meditation. While Patanjali kept descriptions brief, later masters expanded on these steps, eventually shaping what we now recognise as Hatha Yoga – the foundation of most modern Yoga practices.

Hatha Yoga: The Foundation of Therapeutic Yoga

Hatha Yoga focusses on preparing the human body and mind for higher spiritual evolution. It emphasises:

- **Asana** – Works on the physical body, improving flexibility, strength and health.
- **Kriyas** - Cleansing and purification techniques.
- **Pranayama** – Regulates the body's energy systems through breath control.
- **Meditation** – Trains the mind to achieve higher states of awareness.

Over time, Hatha Yoga has been adapted as a therapeutic tool to address imbalances in the body and mind. This integration has led to the development of **Therapeutic Yoga**, which aligns with Naturopathy to form a holistic system of healing: **Naturopathy & Yoga**.

When Yoga is used as a therapeutic method, its spiritual aspect may or may not be considered. Yoga can be seamlessly incorporated into everyone's daily life to achieve health benefits, with or without its spiritual dimension.

Yoga as a Therapeutic Tool

Yoga isn't just about stretching and bending; it's a powerful tool for healing, backed by science and centuries of practice. The beauty of yoga as therapy is that it meets you where you are. You don't need to be flexible, fit or spiritual to benefit from it, just willing to show up for yourself.

Asanas – Healing Through Movement

Asanas, or physical postures, are more than just exercise. They restore balance by improving flexibility, strength and posture. With regular practice, the body feels lighter and more resilient. Movement enhances circulation, aiding the delivery of oxygen and nutrients. It also supports the body's detoxification, promoting overall well-being. Thoughtful practice improves coordination, balance and alignment, laying the foundation for long-term physical health.

Kriyas – Cleansing for Purification and Vitality

Kriyas are yogic cleansing techniques that help the body eliminate toxins and maintain inner harmony. From nasal rinsing to deep intestinal cleansing, each method clears blockages and supports smooth bodily functions. Keeping the body clean from within sharpens the mind, improves energy flow and brings a sense of lightness. Regular practice balances body systems, refines the senses and prepares one for deeper yogic practices. Alongside *asanas*, *pranayama* and meditation, *kriyas* help maintain purity and balance.

Pranayama – The Power of Breath

Pranayama, the art of controlled breathing, greatly influences energy levels and the nervous system. How we breathe affects how we feel.

Conscious breathing relaxes the body and brings mental clarity. Deep, rhythmic breathing creates calm and vitality. Mastering the breath supports emotional balance, making it easier to handle life's challenges with awareness and ease.

Dhyana – Meditation for Mental Clarity and Inner Peace

The mind is always active, processing thoughts and emotions. *Dhyana*, or meditation, helps clear mental clutter and cultivate stillness. It trains the mind to stay present, reduces distractions and deepens awareness. Practiced regularly, it brings clarity, emotional balance and inner peace. It fosters mindfulness and helps create space between thought and reaction, allowing more patient, conscious responses to life.

Bringing It All Together

Yoga as therapy isn't about perfecting poses or chasing enlightenment it's about nurturing both the body and the mind. Simple stretches ease physical tension, mindful breathing restores inner balance and meditation brings mental clarity. These elements work together in harmony, helping the body function at its best. When practiced consistently, yoga becomes a steady support for overall well-being, making each day feel more centred and aligned.

In the chapters ahead I'll be incorporating and detailing these concepts and practices more deeply. Stay tuned.

Naturopathy & Yoga - As the Science of True Healing

When combined together, the philosophy of Naturopathy and Yoga emphasises the intrinsic healing power of the body, rooted in the idea that health is a state of harmony and balance. Here's why Yoga and Naturopathy are vital approaches to health:

- **It is not the absence of medicine, that leads to diseases.**
- **Diseases are the result of broken biochemistry**
- **The body can heal itself, given a chance**

You're Not Just Parts Assembled Together: Embracing Your Wholeness and Completeness

When it comes to health and healing, a holistic approach takes into account the entire person, body, mind and environment, rather than focussing on isolated symptoms.

If you've ever felt that medications only manage the surface level of your issues, you're not alone. Many people are turning to alternative methods because they feel a more comprehensive path, one that sees the whole person, can bring true healing.

Our bodies don't operate in isolated systems; everything is connected. For instance, your gut produces neurotransmitters that influence your brain, which in turn affects your blood chemistry and mood. What's going on in your digestion can shape your thoughts and emotions. Yet the conventional approach often treats the body like a machine, focussing on parts in isolation – like fixing a car without considering how each part interacts with the others.

That's where holism steps in. It recognises that the body is an integrated system where one imbalance can affect the whole. Holistic medicine aims to treat the 'whole person', understanding the dynamic interaction between body, mind and environment. It's not about chasing symptoms; it's about restoring balance and supporting your body's innate intelligence.

In essence, holistic healing sees you as a complete being. It considers how your body, thoughts, emotions and surroundings influence your health and aims to align them to help you feel well and whole.

Holism: The Door to Health and Wellness

Have you ever sensed that your mind and body are more connected than we're often understood? That's the foundation of holism – seeing the big picture in health. It's not about quick fixes or isolated treatments. It's about how your physical, emotional, mental, and even spiritual dimensions work together.

While modern medicine has brought remarkable advances, it sometimes misses the depth of the person behind the symptom. That's why many are embracing holistic medicine – to step back and understand how everything interconnects.

What Is Holism?

Holism is about connection. It acknowledges that every aspect of you - your body, emotions, thoughts, lifestyle and surroundings - are linked. When one part is off, it can ripple through the whole system. The goal is not just to mask symptoms, but to understand the root cause and restore harmony.

Think of your body as an orchestra. If even one instrument is out of tune, the music suffers. Holism is about tuning every part so that the whole can perform beautifully.

Key Principles

1. **Everyone Is Unique:** No two people are exactly alike, so their treatment shouldn't be either. Even with the same condition, two people might respond differently. Your health, genetics, metabolism and gut flora are uniquely yours. Holistic medicine respects this individuality and tailors care accordingly.
2. **Health Is More Than No Illness:** True health isn't just the absence of disease. It's about feeling strong, energetic and balanced, having the resilience to handle life's stressors. Holistic wellness builds this foundation.
3. **Your Body Is Always Adapting:** Your body constantly adjusts to maintain balance in a process called homeodynamics. Like a thermostat regulating temperature, your body fine-tunes itself daily to meet changing conditions. Supporting this adaptability is key to lasting health.
4. **Healing Through Balance:** Instead of fighting disease directly, holism works by supporting the body's natural healing capacity. It's about creating the right conditions for the body to heal itself,

providing rest, nourishment, movement and emotional support, so that the body can do what it's designed to do.

How Does Naturopathy Fit In?

In a reductionist model, the human body is often viewed as a collection of isolated parts. Diseases are labelled based on the organ showing the most distress. But holism invites us to see beyond that.

People often walk into a clinic saying, "I have heart disease," or "My liver is failing." But as a naturopath, I see it differently. You don't have a heart disease or a liver problem, you have a disturbance in the body that's showing up in these organs. Your heart, liver, or kidneys aren't culprits – they're just the victims, saying:

"We've been coping as best we can, but something deeper needs attention. If nothing changes, the whole system will be affected."

Naturopathy and Yoga, as a holistic medical system, has long emphasised treating the whole person. This perspective, rooted in ancient wisdom, is regaining relevance as people recognise the limitations of modern medicine's symptom-focussed approach.

Holism reminds us that lifestyle, mindset and environment are essential to well-being. Naturopathy and Yoga promote living in alignment with nature, supporting the body's own healing intelligence. Instead of forcing the body, we work with it, providing the conditions it needs to restore itself.

Holistic health is empowering. It shifts you from being a passive recipient of treatment to an active participant in your own healing journey. So when your body sends signals – whether pain, fatigue or imbalance – pause and listen. These messages might be your body's way of guiding you back to balance.

Health Beyond Medication: True Healing Starts from Within

"If a doctor prescribes medications without asking about your diet, sleep, stress or exercise, then you didn't meet a doctor - you met a drug dealer."

True healing goes beyond prescriptions. It starts with understanding the root causes and creating space for your body to heal. That's the essence of Naturopathy: to support, not suppress; to build health, not just fight disease.

These statements challenge our typical understanding of health and illness, forcing us to look deeper into the root causes of health issues rather than relying solely on quick fixes. To illustrate this, let me share a story from ancient India.

During the Mughal dynasty, Emperor Akbar challenged his wise minister Birbal to find the biggest fools in the kingdom. As Birbal wandered through a village, he came across a man searching for something under a streetlamp. Curious, Birbal asked, "What are you looking for?"

The man replied, "I lost my ring."

Birbal then asked, "Where did you lose it?"

The man pointed to a dark corner nearby and said, "Over there."

Puzzled, Birbal asked, "Then why are you searching here under the light?"

The man replied, "Because it's easier to see here."

Amused, Birbal realised that he had found the one he was looking for and brought the man to Akbar's court. After narrating the incident, Akbar laughed and asked where the others were. Birbal, with his characteristic wit, replied, "Your Majesty, the other fool is the one who tasked me with finding fools."

This humorous tale carries a profound lesson: people often search for solutions in convenient places rather than addressing the real problem.

Let's connect this to our approach to health. Are you someone who takes a herbal decoction when you experience indigestion, thinking it will solve everything? Though it might have helped, it's worth asking yourself: was indigestion caused by the absence of a herbal decoction? Likely not. The real culprits might be improper food choices, lack of physical activity, poor sleep, high stress levels or a combination of these. Isn't it foolish to believe that a herbal decoction alone can replace the need for a balanced lifestyle?

The decoction might provide temporary relief, but if you continue ignoring the root causes, there will come a time when it stops working. At that point, you may find yourself depending on stronger medications…and the vicious cycle continues. Until and unless you address the underlying issues like diet, activity level, sleep and stress, you cannot achieve true and lasting health.

Are we in essence doing the same thing as the man in Birbal's story? We are losing our health due to poor lifestyle choices, but searching for it in pills and quick remedies. True healing comes from within, from making meaningful and sustainable changes to how we live, eat, move and rest. Only by addressing the root causes can we break free from this cycle and reclaim our well-being.

The Naturopathic Approach: A Logical Hierarchy

Naturopathy offers a wise, structured approach to healing, called the Hierarchy of Therapeutic Intervention. This approach works with the body's natural healing ability, emphasising the use of the least invasive methods first and progressing to more intensive measures only if necessary. Let's explore this step-by-step process:

1. Do Nothing, If Possible: Observation and Rest

The first step is simple: assess whether the body is already beginning to heal. Often, offering rest and simply observing the body's responses is enough. This stage focusses on avoiding unnecessary interference and not overburdening the system. The key idea here is: **don't tax the Vitality,** the healing power within the body.

In Naturopathy, 'vitality' refers to the body's inherent life force, its natural energy that sustains health and drives healing. It is grounded in the belief that the body has its own intelligence and, given the right conditions, can restore balance on its own. Rather than trying to control every symptom, the goal is to support these natural efforts gently and effectively.

Vitality enables the body to maintain homeostasis, repair damage and respond to challenges. This vital force underlies all biological processes and ensures overall functioning. Two guiding principles here are the **law of minimum** – intervene only as much as necessary – and the **conservation of energy**, which highlights the healing value of rest. Overstimulating the system, even with natural therapies, can drain this energy and slow down recovery.

Symptoms like fever, inflammation or pain are seen not as enemies, but as signs that the vital force is actively working. Suppressing them can interfere with healing. Instead, Naturopathy encourages us to reduce the total burden on the system through rest, proper hydration and nutrition, allowing these signs to guide our care, not silence them.

Modern science supports this view. Vitality aligns with **Bioenergetics**, which looks at how cells create and use energy for repair and growth. **Homeostasis**, a fundamental concept in physiology, mirrors this idea, showing how the body constantly adapts to maintain internal balance. The work of **Hans Selye** on stress (General Adaptation Syndrome) describes how the body mobilises energy to cope with challenges – a modern parallel to the concept of vitality.

Research in **Sleep Science** also confirms the regenerative power of rest. During sleep, the body repairs tissues, strengthens immunity and clears toxins from the brain via the lymphatic system. Similarly, studies in **Psychoneuroimmunology** show that over-treatment or excessive intervention can increase stress and disrupt healing*.

These findings support the naturopathic wisdom of stepping back and letting the body do its work.

In practice, this means starting with rest and observation. Before offering any treatment, practitioners must consider whether the individual has enough energy to respond well. Even gentle therapies like massage, fasting or hydrotherapy can strain the system if applied without assessing the person's vitality.

Hans Selye's General Adaptation Syndrome (GAS)

Hans Selye's General Adaptation Syndrome (GAS) describes the body's predictable, multi-phase response to prolonged stress, encompassing three stages:

- Alarm, where the body activates the fight-or-flight response through stress hormones like adrenaline and cortisol.
- Resistance, where the body attempts to adapt to the stressor while maintaining heightened physiological function.
- Exhaustion, where prolonged stress depletes the body's resources, leading to fatigue, weakened immunity and vulnerability to illness.

Selye's framework highlights the impact of chronic stress on health, linking it to conditions like cardiovascular disease and depression, and emphasises the importance of stress management to prevent exhaustion. His work laid the foundation for understanding stress physiology and its interplay with health, contributing to fields like Psychoneuroimmunology. *(Selye, 1956).*

---

* (Kiecolt-Glaser, J. K., Marucha, P. T., Mercado, A. M., Malarkey, W. B., & Glaser, R. (1995). **Slowing of wound healing by psychological stress**. *The Lancet, 346*(8984), 1194–1196. https://doi.org/10.1016/S0140-6736(95)92899-5)

Naturopathy's concept of vitality elegantly bridges ancient wisdom and modern biology. By supporting rather than pushing the body, we create space for true healing. Sometimes, the best approach is patience, presence and trust in the body's inner intelligence. That's the essence of 'Do Nothing, If Possible', letting nature lead the way when it's already doing the work.

2. Establish Optimum Conditions for Healing

While rest and observation form the foundation, sometimes 'doing nothing' isn't enough. If the environment remains toxic or imbalanced, the causes of illness may persist or even worsen.

The principle, *"You can never get healed in the same environment that you got diseased"* highlights the need to transform the very conditions that contributed to the illness. This includes shifting both internal and external influences.

Internally, factors like diet, emotional stress and mental strain can introduce toxins that block healing. It's not just physical detox that matters; unresolved emotional stress and negative thought patterns create a toxic inner world that undermines recovery. Practices like mindfulness, meditation and emotional release work to clear these blocks, giving the body the mental space to begin healing.

Externally, environmental toxins such as pollutants, chemicals and electromagnetic radiation can interfere with the healing process. Creating a toxin-free home, improving air quality and switching to natural products can help remove these obstacles. Connecting with nature through practices like 'earthing' helps rebalance the body, reduce inflammation and support circulation. Limiting exposure to unhealthy relationships, environmental stressors and toxic surroundings is equally important. Together, these adjustments help create a healing-friendly atmosphere.

By removing what hinders healing – be it poor food choices, stress or toxic environments – and creating conditions that nurture balance and restoration, we realign the body with its natural rhythm. This isn't just about recovering from illness; it's about moving towards a way of living that fosters vitality and resilience.

The goal is simple: replace what harms with what heals. When both the internal and external environments are aligned to support health, the body is empowered to do what it does best: heal and thrive.

3. Stimulate and Assist the Body's Self-Healing Power

If lifestyle changes alone are insufficient to address the underlying imbalances, the focus shifts to stimulating the body's inherent healing mechanisms using targeted techniques. This approach aligns with the naturopathic principle of treating the whole body, recognising that disease occurs within the body but manifests in specific organs or systems. Therefore, the primary goal is to support and enhance the body's natural healing power through generalised treatments that address systemic health rather than isolated symptoms.

These treatments include therapeutic massages, which help improve circulation, relieve muscular tension and promote relaxation. Yoga therapy plays a pivotal role, incorporating *pranayama* (breathing exercises) to enhance oxygenation, calm the nervous system and balance energy, alongside *asanas* (postures) that foster physical and mental equilibrium. Naturopathic interventions such as hydrotherapy are used to detoxify and rejuvenate the body through the application of water at varying temperatures and pressures. Additionally, fasting or juice therapy may be used to provide the digestive system with rest, allowing the body to channel energy toward repair and regeneration.

This stage of treatment is typically implemented under the guidance of a qualified Yoga Naturopathy doctor in a clinical setting, ensuring safety and efficacy. The ultimate goal is to enhance the body's ability to repair itself, restore balance and achieve optimal health holistically, addressing both the root causes and the systemic manifestations of disease.

4. Support Specific Weak or Damaged Organs

When the body is too weak or damaged to heal certain areas on its own, more targeted and specific interventions become necessary. While a holistic approach views the body as a whole, focussed support can be crucial when specific dysfunctions – especially those causing pain – hinder the body's ability to recover naturally. Supportive measures may include herbal medicines for specific organs, dietary changes to restore nutrients and probiotics or enzymes to aid digestion and absorption. Pain management therapies like topical herbal applications, acupuncture and acupressure can help reduce discomfort, allowing healing energy to flow where it's needed.

Nutraceuticals are a valuable tool in this process. These bioactive compounds, naturally found in food, go beyond basic nutrition to strengthen weak systems and help prevent disease. Acting as a bridge between food and medicine, nutraceuticals align with the body's natural processes. Naturopathy embraces them as gentle yet effective tools to support organ function and restore balance. Unlike synthetic supplements, which can sometimes burden the system, nutraceuticals – derived from whole foods – are more easily absorbed and work harmoniously with the body.

That said, they must be used with discernment and never replace the foundation of a whole-food, nutrient-rich diet. While they provide targeted support, the real healing still depends on consistently nourishing the body with real food. Some humorously call this approach 'Green Allopathy', a reminder to use even natural remedies with mindfulness and care.

Therapeutic yoga and specific *pranayama* techniques also play a key role in supporting weakened systems, especially the lungs. These practices build strength, enhance flexibility, improve oxygen flow and reduce stress, creating favourable conditions for healing.

Ultimately, these interventions do more than just relieve symptoms; they help sustain the patient's confidence and hope. Pain relief and symptom management are crucial for emotional and mental well-being, both of which are central to recovery. By offering targeted support where it's needed most while honouring the body's wholeness, we create a healing environment where function can be restored and overall balance maintained.

5. Address Pathology with Medications or Surgery

In cases where previous measures are insufficient, the focus shifts to directly addressing the underlying pathology through medications or surgery. This may involve the use of pharmaceutical drugs, advanced therapies, or surgical procedures to ensure patient safety and prevent further harm. At this stage, the goal is to stabilise the condition and minimise any disruption to the body's natural processes. It is crucial to make this decision at the right time, with the understanding that saving the patient's life is of utmost importance, even if more invasive interventions are necessary. A naturopath, not trained in such interventions, should not attempt to address conditions that require medications or surgery. It is important to seek the help of medical experts when such situations arise, as they are equipped to manage the pathology directly and ensure patient safety. The decision to pursue these interventions should be made carefully and at the right time, always prioritising preservation of the patient's life.

A Balanced Perspective on Healing

This hierarchy demonstrates that all available methods of healing, including medication, have their place. The key is to use them in the right order, starting with the least invasive approaches. It ensures that the patient's natural healing capacity is supported and strengthened rather than bypassed or suppressed, providing a sustainable pathway to health. Unfortunately, many people reverse this process, reaching for pills first and only turning to holistic methods when the damage has worsened. This backward approach often results in deeper harm, reinforcing the age-old wisdom: 'A stitch in time saves nine'.

Guiding Principles of This Approach

1. Minimal Intervention: Start with the least invasive, least disruptive methods.
2. Root Cause Focus: Address the origin of the illness, not just the symptoms.
3. Empowering the Patient: Encourage the patient's active participation in the healing process.
4. Whole-Person Healing: Consider physical, emotional and spiritual aspects at every stage.

When converting this approach into practice, is it important that the Naturopathy physician follows the Step-by-Step Process

1. Comprehensive Assessment: Begin with a detailed history and physical examination, including questions about lifestyle, diet, stress and emotional health.
2. Identify Root Causes: Use a holistic framework to pinpoint both the first cause and current contributors.
3. Personalised Plan: Develop a treatment plan that addresses the patient's unique needs, starting with the least invasive therapies.
4. Ongoing Support: Monitor progress and make adjustments based on the patient's response.
5. Patient Empowerment: Equip the patient with the tools and knowledge to sustain their health long-term.

While medications may have their place, they will never replace the importance of a healthy lifestyle. As the quotes remind us, diseases don't develop because we didn't take a pill; they arise when we fail to take care of our bodies and minds. By embracing a holistic approach to health, we empower ourselves to heal and thrive in a way that goes far beyond any prescription.

If the body has the ability to heal itself, then what is the role of a Yoga and Naturopathy physician?

One of the fundamental principles of Naturopathy is that a doctor is not just a healer but also a teacher. Healing is not about simply prescribing remedies; it's about guiding people to take charge of their own health. My role as a Yoga and Naturopathy physician is to empower individuals to make informed decisions, set realistic health goals, and bring balance and consistency into their lives. I help people navigate their healing journey by understanding the deeper causes of their health concerns, rather than just addressing symptoms.

Let me walk you through the steps of how we'll approach your healing together:

1. What is the First Cause?

To begin, we need to understand what started this whole process. There are many factors that could have contributed to your health issue, and we'll look at everything. This might include:

- Lifestyle Factors: Are there issues with your diet, exercise routine, sleep or stress management?
- Environmental Factors: Have you been exposed to toxins, pollutants or allergens?
- Genetic Factors: Are there family health patterns or inherited susceptibilities we should be aware of?
- Past Medical History: Have previous illnesses, treatments or traumas disrupted your body's balance?

2. What Is Contributing Now?

Next, we'll explore what's currently making things worse or preventing your body from healing. This includes:

- Ongoing Stress: Are there emotional, physical or psychological stresses that are impacting your health?

- Habits: Are there any nutritional gaps, unhealthy behaviours or coping mechanisms that might be affecting you?
- Current Environment: Do work, relationships or living conditions play a role in your health?
- Medical Treatments: Are any of your current medications or treatments just managing symptoms instead of addressing the root cause?

3. How Is Your Body Trying to Heal Itself?

The body has an incredible ability to repair and restore itself. Our job is to recognise how it's already trying to heal. This might show up as:

- Signs of Compensation: For example, inflammation or a mild fever could be your body's way of defending itself.
- Self-regulation: Your hormones, digestive system or nervous system might be adjusting on their own to help you recover.
- Areas of Strength: Let's also look for areas where your body is strong and resilient. These are things we can support to help your overall healing.

4. What's the Minimum Intervention Needed?

In Naturopathy & Yoga we follow the principle of 'do no harm'. That means we start with the least invasive methods by removing obstacles in the path of healing and using gentle interventions to begin with.

5. What Are Your Underlying Weaknesses?

Let's take a closer look at the areas where your body might be struggling. We'll focus on:

- Digestion: Are you having trouble absorbing nutrients or dealing with digestive issues?

- Detoxification: Is your body's ability to detoxify (like the liver or kidneys) functioning properly?
- Hormonal Balance: Are there any imbalances in your hormones or immune system?
- Structural Issues: Do you have any misalignments or tension in your body that might affect your overall health?

6. What Education Do You Need?

It's important that you understand your health journey and how you can support it. I'll help you learn about:

- The root causes of your condition and how they developed over time.
- The connection between lifestyle, diet, stress and health – it's all interconnected!
- Actionable steps you can take every day to support your healing process.
- The importance of a holistic approach, focussing on long-term health rather than relying on quick fixes.

7. How Does Your Physical Health Relate to Your Emotional and Spiritual Well-Being?

In Yoga and Naturopathy we believe that the mind, body and spirit are deeply connected. So we'll also explore:

- Psychological Factors: Is stress, anxiety, unresolved trauma or negative thinking showing up as physical symptoms in your body?
- Spiritual Health: Do you feel a sense of purpose, peace and connection in your life?
- Mind-body Practices: We can use tools like meditation, mindfulness and breathing exercises to address both your emotional and physical health.

So far, we've been navigating through the various concepts of health and healing – the foundational principles of holistic well-being and the core approach of Naturopathy & Yoga.

Now comes the exciting part, the moment where we take everything we've explored and begin to put it into practice.

Together we'll start uncovering what's been throwing your system off balance and make simple, natural adjustments to support your body's innate ability to heal. Yes, it takes time, but with the right approach and a little patience, healing is absolutely within your reach.

At the heart of it all, true healing is about working with nature, not against it.

After all, *knowing without doing is the same as not knowing at all.*

So how do we actually do it? How do we move from knowledge to action?

Welcome to the next leg of your journey, the part where healing truly begins!

"The greatest medicine of all is to teach people how not to need it."

Bringing Back the Balance: The Power of DRAMMER

Let's begin the most exciting part of the journey, that I promised you in the beginning - Awakening the Healer in You, awakening and assisting your own body to get healed, to be healthy.

Healing is all about bringing back the balance. How do we do it? Is there any *mantra*? Any shortcuts? Yes, there is a *mantra*: **DRAMMER**. But this is not to chant, it's to practice, because there are no shortcuts. This journey we are committed to is not for the person who always look for links like '7 Easy Steps to Reduce Tummy Fat' or 'The Superfood That Removes Cholesterol and Blocks in the Heart'. Let me make it clear before we proceed: short-term plans or responses will never help you attain long-term goals or sustainable results.

When it comes to true healing and lasting health, balance is everything. But how do you actually bring that balance back? This is where DRAMMER comes in.

Take a moment. What could it stand for? Think about the key elements of life that nourish and sustain you. Is it about food? Movement? Maybe something deeper?

DRAMMER is an acronym for

D - Diet
R - Rest
A - Activity
M - Mind
M - Microbiome
E - Elements
R - Rhythm.

These are not just words; they are the holistic foundation of health and healing from a naturopathic perspective.

Each of these elements plays a crucial role, and none of them work in isolation. Think about it – Diet is not just about what you eat, but how it affects your gut Microbiome and quality of Rest. Rest doesn't

Bringing Back the Balance: The Power of DRAMMER (*contd.*)

just mean sleep; it rejuvenates the Mind and balances gut health. Exercise? It's more than just movement; it influences your diet choices, body Rhythm and overall vitality. Your Environment shapes your well-being in ways you may not even realise. Everything is deeply interconnected, like a web holding your health together. Ignore one, and the whole system feels the impact.

For example, you can eat the most nutrient-dense foods, but if your sleep is poor and your stress levels are high, your body won't fully absorb and utilise those nutrients. You might have a great exercise routine, but if your gut microbiome is imbalanced, your energy and recovery will suffer. It's all about creating harmony among these elements.

DRAMMER is not just a framework, it's a reminder that your body thrives when everything works together. The goal is not perfection, but integration. When you start looking at health from this holistic perspective, you create the conditions for deep, natural healing and long-term well-being.

Now it's time to dive deeper. Each of these elements holds a wealth of insight, hidden connections and fascinating science that can transform the way you approach your health. As you continue this journey, you'll uncover how.

What you're about to discover may change the way you see health forever.

CHAPTER 3

The Communication

Diet: The 'Why' Is What Matters!

I can't count how many times people have approached me not only in the clinic, but also at family gatherings, parties or even during casual conversation, asking the same question:

"I have diabetes... I am obese... I have heart issues...
What should I eat?"

Let me be honest: I've never had a perfect answer to this. Not because I don't know about food or health, but because the question itself is not the right one to ask.

When people ask *what* to eat, they are looking for a quick-fix solution, like a pill that can magically control their blood sugar, weight or heart health. But food doesn't work that way. It *can't* work that way.

So what should be the right question?

I believe it should be: **"Why should I eat?"**

Whenever I ask this question in my classes or discussions, the answers are usually straightforward: "To get energy." "To get nutrition." "To stay alive."

And then I throw their own answers back at them: *When was the last time you ate because your body was truly deprived of nutrients? When was the last time you ate because you were at the edge of starvation?*

Most people pause. Because in reality, we don't eat for these reasons.

We eat because the clock tells us it's lunchtime.

We eat because someone offered us food.

We eat because we saw something delicious on the table.

We eat for pleasure, entertainment or emotional reasons, when we're stressed, bored or upset.

This reveals something very important: food is more than just fuel for the body**; food is a conversation, a communication** between the world outside and the cells inside us.

Just as **disease is the body's way of communicating with us, food is how we communicate back.**

If this communication is clear and aligned with what our body truly needs, we stay healthy. If it is distorted, if we eat for the wrong reasons, without awareness, it leads to disorder and disease.

Think about it – every bite of food carries a message. The sun, the soil, the rain, the plants, the animals, the honeybee all play a role in bringing that food to our plate. And when we eat, we are not just consuming calories, we are receiving information from all these. These information influences how our cells function, how our metabolism works and how our body heals or breaks down over time. Food influences our physical health as well as emotional well-being. By eating with intention and mindfulness, we can ensure that the communication between our external environment and our internal body is positive. This promotes healing, energy and emotional stability. Making conscious food choices ensures that the messages our body receives contribute to optimal health and harmony

So, the real question is not *"What should I eat?"* but rather, *"What kind of message do I want to send to my body?"*

In the next section, we will explore the basic principles of eating in a way that supports health and healing: How to ensure that every meal we take is sending the right message to our body.

Principles of Eating: A Naturopathic Perspective

Eat Your Liquids, Drink Your Solids

The principle of 'eat your liquids, drink your solids' highlights the importance of mindful eating and proper digestion. Liquids, such as soups, broths or smoothies should be sipped slowly rather than gulped down. This allows the liquid to mix with saliva in the mouth, where enzymes like amylase begin the digestion of carbohydrates. Saliva also contains other beneficial compounds, such as mucin, which helps protect the digestive tract. By thoroughly engaging with liquids in this way, the body can better prepare them for the next stages of digestion, ensuring improved nutrient absorption and reduced strain on the digestive system.

Similarly, solid foods should be chewed thoroughly until they reach an almost liquid consistency. This mechanical breakdown not only reduces the digestive workload on the stomach, but also increases the surface area for digestive enzymes to act upon. Chewing activates salivary glands, releasing enzymes that start carbohydrate digestion while signalling the stomach to release hydrochloric acid for protein breakdown. This process enhances enzymatic activity, improves nutrient extraction and promotes gut health. By chewing solids and sipping liquids mindfully, the body can work more efficiently, leading to improved digestion, better absorption of nutrients and a healthier gastrointestinal system.

Food is Not Medicine; Food is Just Food

Food plays a vital role in nourishing the body and maintaining balance, but it is not a substitute for targeted medical treatments or medications. Viewing food solely as a tool for healing can place undue pressure on dietary choices, potentially leading to stress and an unhealthy relationship with eating. While food supports the body's innate ability to heal and maintain health, it is only one element of holistic well-being. Healing requires a broader approach, incorporating rest, movement, emotional well-being and, when necessary, appropriate medical care. By understanding food as nourishment rather than a 'cure', individuals can develop a more natural, relaxed relationship with their diet.

When food is seen as medicine, it may lead to forced consumption of foods one dislikes, potentially causing emotional stress. This stress can counteract the intended health benefits of the food, as emotional strain impacts digestion and overall well-being. Conversely, enjoying the foods you eat fosters a sense of satisfaction and comfort, reducing stress and allowing the body to process nutrients more effectively. While food is not a substitute for medication, it can help prevent the need for medication by promoting long-term health through balanced nutrition. A mindful approach to eating – focussed on enjoyment and nourishment – encourages a positive relationship with food and supports overall health without making food the sole focus of healing.

Listen to Your Body; It Knows How Much to Eat

Listen to Cellular Intelligence: Our bodies are equipped with remarkable intelligence at the cellular level, a wisdom that guides us toward health and well-being. This cellular intelligence is not just a concept, but a living, breathing process that governs every aspect of our biological functions. From the way our cells communicate with each other to how they respond to external stimuli, the body's innate wisdom orchestrates the balance necessary for vitality and healing. Listening to this cellular intelligence involves tuning into the subtle signals of our body: hunger, fatigue, cravings and even emotions that are often influenced by the intricate processes within our cells. By fostering an awareness of these signals and honouring the body's natural rhythms, we align ourselves with our own health, ensuring that we nourish and support the body's innate ability to maintain balance. This mindful approach to listening and responding to cellular intelligence offers a pathway to a healthier, more harmonious life.

When it comes to eating, the body has an innate ability to regulate food intake through complex hormonal signals, primarily mediated by ghrelin and leptin. Ghrelin, often referred to as the 'hunger hormone', signals the brain when it's time to eat, triggering the familiar growl of hunger. Conversely, leptin, known as the 'satiety hormone', tells the body when it has had enough food. These hormones work together to maintain a delicate balance, ensuring that the body receives the right amount of nourishment. This system operates optimally when one follows a natural, balanced diet, allowing the body to effectively gauge hunger and fullness.

However, when the body is subjected to an unhealthy diet often rich in processed foods or lacking essential nutrients, this hormonal communication can become disrupted. Inflammation from poor dietary choices can lead to resistance to leptin and ghrelin, causing the body to either overeat or under-eat. Leptin resistance, for example, may prevent the body from recognising when it is full, while ghrelin may increase hunger signals excessively. This cycle of inflammation and hormonal resistance contributes to overeating, weight gain and metabolic disorders, creating a vicious cycle. By listening to and respecting the body's natural hunger cues through a whole nutrient-dense diet, we can support the natural regulatory systems and prevent these imbalances from occurring.

Food Should Be Friendly to Digest, Not Easy to Digest

The concept of 'digestive-friendly food' emphasises the importance of foods that encourage the natural activation of digestive enzymes, rather than foods that are too easy to digest. Much like cooking with fire, where we avoid using paper (which burns too quickly and doesn't provide sustained heat) in favour of wood (which burns more steadily), our bodies benefit from foods that require some effort to digest, but in a way that supports long-term digestive health. Foods rich in fibre, natural enzymes and balanced nutrients engage the digestive system, helping to stimulate and strengthen the organs involved in digestion, such as the stomach and intestines. In contrast, overly processed foods that are too 'easy' to digest – often stripped of fibre and nutrients – can weaken the digestive system over time, leading to issues like sluggish digestion and nutrient deficiencies.

Digestive-friendly foods work in harmony with our body's natural processes, aiding in the gradual and sustainable release of energy and nutrients. By encouraging slow and steady digestion, these foods help maintain balanced blood sugar levels, preventing energy spikes and crashes that can occur with overly processed foods. Much like firewood providing steady heat, foods that require some effort to digest contribute to the steady burning of energy in the body, promoting stable energy levels throughout the day and better overall health. The key is to focus on whole, nutrient-dense foods that nourish and support the digestive system, rather than opting for quick, overly processed foods that may disrupt the body's natural balance.

Food Should Attract You: A Natural Connection

In Naturopathy, the attraction to food is viewed as an intuitive, biological response to the body's nutritional needs. Just like animals are naturally drawn to their instinctive foods – goats to grass or lions to rabbits – humans have an innate attraction to foods that will nourish them. This attraction is a reflection of the body's wisdom, signalling to us which foods will support our health at any given moment. This connection is not just physical, but also psychological and emotional, as we tend to crave the foods that our bodies need for balance and healing.

Consider the example of a mango: When it ripens, it naturally emits a fragrance, changes colour and falls from the tree. These transformations are designed to attract animals (and humans) to consume the fruit. By eating the mango, we not only enjoy its sweet, nourishing flesh, but also help the tree fulfil its purpose of dispersing seeds. The mango tree benefits from this process as its offspring – new trees – are spread far and wide. Similarly, our attraction to naturally ripened, wholesome foods is not coincidental; it is part of a mutually beneficial, natural cycle where both the food and the eater are nourished. Just as the mango uses its vibrant colour and aroma to draw us in, our body is naturally inclined to seek the nourishment that aligns with its needs, reinforcing the deep connection between humans and nature's bounty.

Digestion Starts from the Brain; Eat with Your Senses

Digestion is not solely a physical process that begins in the stomach; it actually starts in the brain. Many people think that the only way to judge food is by its taste, but digestion begins long before food reaches your mouth. As soon as you see, smell or even think about food, your brain activates the digestive process. This sensory perception triggers the release of saliva and digestive enzymes, preparing your body to break down the food efficiently. Eating in a calm, pleasant environment enhances this brain-body connection, promoting relaxation, reducing stress and improving the overall digestive process.

Eating is a multi-sensory experience that goes beyond just tasting food. At Prakriti Shakti, we emphasise the importance of engaging all the senses when eating. We encourage patients to:

1. Hear about the food: Listen to the sounds of food being prepared, served or even chewed, which can increase anticipation and enhance enjoyment.
2. Smell its aroma: The smell of food plays a crucial role in stimulating the digestive system and increasing salivation.
3. See and appreciate its visual appeal: The sight of food, especially when vibrant and well-presented, signals the brain that nourishment is coming.
4. Touch and feel its texture: The texture of food – whether smooth, crunchy or chewy – adds to the overall sensory experience and satisfaction.
5. Finally, taste and savour it: The act of tasting should be a mindful and enjoyable process, allowing the full range of flavours to unfold.

This holistic, mindful approach to eating ensures that food nourishes both the body and mind. We encourage patients to only eat what they truly enjoy, recognising that food is not medicine and should never be forced upon the body. By embracing the full sensory experience of eating, we create a deeper connection to the food we consume and promote optimal digestion and overall well-being.

Gut is the Second Brain

What you are, how you think, and how you feel are all deeply influenced by the health of your gut. The concept of a 'gut feeling' is not just an intuitive sense; it is a direct reflection of how your gut interacts with external factors and communicates with the brain. The gut houses its own neural network, known as the enteric nervous system, which is responsible for regulating digestion and managing signals to the brain. This complex system has the ability to influence your thoughts, emotions and physical state, making it clear that your gut is not just about digestion, but a key player in your mental and emotional health.

The health of your gut microbiome, the collection of bacteria and other microorganisms in the digestive system, is crucial for overall well-being. A balanced, thriving microbiome supports mental clarity, emotional stability and physical health. Naturopathy focuses on nourishing the gut with natural, whole foods that support a healthy microbiome. By incorporating prebiotics, which feed beneficial bacteria, and probiotics, which introduce good bacteria into the gut, we can maintain a harmonious gut-brain connection. In this way, gut health is central to achieving optimal health, helping us think clearer, feel balanced and maintain physical vitality.

Know Hunger, Not Appetite

Hunger and appetite are often mistaken for one another, but they are fundamentally different. Hunger is the body's natural signal that it requires nourishment to sustain itself. It is a biological mechanism, deeply rooted in survival instincts, ensuring that the body obtains the necessary energy and nutrients to function optimally. Unlike appetite, which can be influenced by external cues like emotions or environmental triggers, hunger is a purely physiological response.

Take the example of a lion looking for food after a period of fasting. In the wild, fasting is a natural part of a predator's life, as they do not have consistent access to prey. If hunger caused the lion to feel weak or lethargic during this period, it would spell disaster. A weak lion cannot chase a fast-moving deer or rabbit, and without the strength to hunt it would fail to secure its next meal, eventually leading to its death.

However, nature has designed hunger differently for such scenarios. When a lion fasts, its body adapts to ensure survival. Instead of becoming tired, the lion enters a heightened state of focus and energy when it feels hungry. This is because the body releases hormones, such as adrenaline and norepinephrine, during fasting. These hormones stimulate alertness, enhance physical performance and sharpen the lion's hunting instincts. The lion becomes more agile and mentally concentrated, enabling it to outrun and outmanoeuvre the prey that is naturally faster or more evasive.

Similarly, in humans, the body operates with intelligence to signal when it is time to break the fast. As the fasting process nears its natural conclusion, the person does not feel weak or drained, but experiences a surge of energy and focus. This is accompanied by a genuine and pleasant sensation of hunger – a signal that the body is now ready to receive nourishment. This hunger is distinct from the cravings driven by appetite; it is clear, purposeful and deeply satisfying.

This physiological response ensures that fasting ends at the right moment, when the body has completed its restorative processes and is prepared to resume normal nourishment. Just as the lion feels energised and focussed to secure its prey, the person breaking a therapeutic fast feels revitalised and attuned to the body's genuine need for food, making the experience both natural and harmonious.

Recognising the difference between hunger and appetite is key to mindful eating. When we listen to true hunger, we eat to fulfil the body's nutritional requirements, which helps maintain balance and health. In contrast, eating driven by appetite – especially when we're not truly hungry – can lead to overeating, strain the digestive system and disrupt the body's natural processes. By tuning into real hunger signals, we can align our eating habits with the body's actual needs, fostering better digestion and preventing unnecessary strain on the system.

Eat One Portion Less Than You Can: A Path to Balance and Health

In the modern world, overeating has become a common issue, placing unnecessary strain on the digestive system and leading to a range of metabolic imbalances, sluggishness and poor nutrient absorption. Naturopathy emphasises the principle of moderation in eating, teaching us that eating in a way that supports the body's natural rhythm is essential for maintaining good health. By consuming just one portion less than we think we can eat, we allow space for efficient digestion and proper nutrient absorption, preventing digestive distress and helping to maintain optimal energy levels throughout the day.

This principle is deeply rooted in the yogic tradition, where moderation in eating is viewed as crucial for both physical and spiritual well-being. The saying '*Ekabhuktham mahayogi, dwibhuktam mahabhogi, thribhuktam maharogi'* translates to:

- '*Ekabhuktham Mahayogi*: 'The one who eats once is a great yogi'. This highlights the yogi's discipline in eating only when necessary, focussing on spiritual growth and balance rather than indulgence.
- '*Dwibhuktam Mahabhogi*': 'The one who eats twice is a hedonist'. This suggests that those who indulge in food more than once a day risk falling into excessive enjoyment and losing sight of balance, leading to a pleasure-driven approach to eating.
- '*Thribhuktam Maharogi'*: 'The one who eats three times becomes diseased'. This part warns that eating too frequently or in excess

can lead to digestive issues, metabolic problems and disease. Overeating taxes the digestive system, leading to imbalance and poor health.

The yogic wisdom in this saying underscores the importance of mindfulness and moderation in eating. By eating only when necessary and consuming less than our full capacity, we create space for the body to digest food properly and maintain balance. This aligns with the concept of *Mithahara* in Hatha Yoga, which translates to 'moderate eating'. The practice of *Mithahara* is not just about physical moderation, but about fostering awareness and aligning eating habits with the body's natural needs.

Ultimately, eating one portion less than we can is a practice that not only supports the physical digestive process, but also promotes mental clarity, emotional stability and spiritual growth. By cultivating awareness of our hunger and eating mindfully, we honour our body's natural capacity for digestion and nourishment, leading to a healthier, more balanced life.

Eat with Gratitude – *Annadata Sukhibhava*

Eating with gratitude strengthens our connection to the food we consume and the natural world. In yogic and naturopathic traditions, gratitude for food goes beyond appreciating its taste or appearance. The phrase '*Annadata Sukhibhava*' translates to 'May the provider of food be happy'. This extends beyond just thanking the cook to recognising the collective effort and resources that bring food to our table. It acknowledges the sun, soil, rain, bees, farmers, traders and cooks who play a part in the nourishment we receive.

By practicing gratitude for food, we cultivate mindfulness, fostering respect for the Earth and all beings involved in the food process. This holistic view of food emphasises the interconnectedness of nature and humanity, encouraging us to honour the environment and the labour behind our meals.

This practice transforms eating into a mindful, sacred act, promoting better digestion and overall well-being. It encourages us to be conscious of the preciousness of our food, enhancing the experience of nourishment and helping us align with the natural cycles that sustain us.

Chewing is the First Step of Digestion

Chewing plays a crucial role in the digestive process, acting as the first step in breaking down food. By thoroughly chewing, we mechanically break down the food into smaller pieces, which increases its surface area and prepares it for enzymatic action in the stomach. This process ensures that food enters the stomach in an optimal state, reducing the chances of bloating, gas or indigestion. When food isn't properly chewed, it's akin to passing an unfinished product to the next stage in a process, which can disrupt efficient digestion and nutrient absorption.

Chewing also offers additional health benefits. It acts as a natural exercise for the jaw, strengthening the jawbones and facial muscles. A strong jaw contributes to maintaining the structure of the face and neck, preventing sagging, which is one of the most visible signs of ageing. Weak jaw muscles can lead to a lack of facial tone, making proper chewing an anti-ageing practice as well. By dedicating time to chew food thoroughly, we support both our digestive health and facial muscle strength, promoting a more youthful and vibrant appearance.

Food is the Greatest Addiction

In the grand tapestry of life, food serves not just as nourishment, but as a symbol of connection, celebration and survival. Yet, in the modern world, it has transformed from a simple source of sustenance to something far more complex – an emotional crutch, a source of comfort and at times, a source of addiction. We often overlook the profound relationship we have with food, one that begins the moment we are born and continues to shape our experiences and well-being. In this complex dance with food, the question arises: Are we truly in control, or have we allowed food to control us?

Food addiction often stems from emotional associations, cravings or a dependence on processed foods. Since eating is something we do multiple times a day, often beginning at birth, food becomes deeply intertwined with many aspects of our lives – celebrations, emotions, social gatherings and daily habits. For some, food serves as a stress reliever; for others, it's a way to pass time; and for many, it becomes a source of pleasure. This emotional connection can turn food into a temptation, making it difficult to say no, especially when it is readily available or offered.

Naturopathy encourages breaking free from this cycle by resetting the palate and focussing on natural, whole foods. By developing a mindful approach to eating and fostering a balanced relationship with food, we can learn to recognise when we are eating out of habit or emotion rather than true hunger. Part of this journey is learning to say 'No' or 'Enough' when necessary. Overcoming food addiction is an important step in cultivating healthy dietary habits and taking control of our relationship with food.

It is Better to Waste Outside, than Inside

From childhood, we have often heard, "Don't waste food, eat everything on your plate – people are starving." While the sentiment comes from a place of compassion, we must ask ourselves: Has overeating to avoid food waste ever truly solved the problem of world hunger? The truth is, forcing ourselves to eat more than necessary simply to avoid waste does not help anyone. In fact, it can harm our health and well-being.

Overeating stresses the digestive system, making it work harder to process unnecessary food. This can lead to indigestion, bloating, toxicity or even fat accumulation. Instead of overloading the body, we can choose to take less on our plate, being mindful of our true hunger. If there is food left over, it is better to waste it outside, rather than putting unnecessary strain on our body by consuming beyond its capacity. This approach promotes a healthier, more conscious relationship with food, allowing us to honour both our body's needs and the global reality of food scarcity.

Be a 'Vegetablarian' - Not Vegetarian

People often tell me with a puzzled expression, "I don't know where I went wrong. I am a pure vegetarian, yet I suffer from lifestyle disorders." This confusion stems from the belief that simply avoiding meat ensures good health, but that's far from the truth. All kinds of processed, unhealthy foods that contribute to nutritional deficiencies and chronic diseases can be part of the diet of a pure vegetarian. That's why I introduce the term **'Vegetablarian',** to emphasise the difference between merely being vegetarian and actually prioritising vegetables as the foundation of one's diet. Vegetables are nature's true healing foods, packed with essential vitamins, minerals, fibre and antioxidants that nourish the body at a cellular level. They promote gut health, regulate blood sugar, enhance immunity, support detoxification and help prevent lifestyle diseases. A true **Vegetablarian** ensures that at least 50 percent of their daily intake consists of vegetables, making them a staple rather than an afterthought. A simple yet powerful shift – one meal a day made entirely of vegetables, a plate full of salad before indulging in other foods or a conscious effort to fill the plate with more colours from nature – can transform health in profound ways. Being a **Vegetablarian** is not about exclusion; it's about abundance, the abundance of real, life-giving food that restores balance, vitality and longevity.

Therapeutic Diet - Naturopathic Approach

Therapeutic diet prescription in Naturopathy aligns with its core principles, primarily the elimination of toxic matter from the body and supporting the body's efforts to restore balance.

Classification of Diet in Naturopathy

If you are undergoing a healing programme as an inpatient in a Naturopathy hospital, you may go through different stages of a therapeutic diet. Naturopathy categorises diet into three stages:

1. **Constructive Stage**
2. **Soothing Stage**
3. **Eliminative Stage**

During naturopathic treatment, a patient undergoes these three phases sequentially, with an appropriate diet prescribed at each stage.

Constructive Stage

This is the healthy diet phase, which provides nourishment to the body. When a person is admitted to a Naturopathy hospital, they might start with a constructive diet, gradually shifting to a soothing diet and then finally to an eliminative diet. Once the cleansing is complete, they will be transitioned back to the constructive phase through the soothing stage once again.

The constructive phase emphasises a balanced diet free from processed and unhealthy foods, such as oils, refined flour (*maida*), sugar, fast foods and bakery items. Instead, the focus is on whole, natural foods, including sprouts, salads and nutrient-dense meals that provide essential energy for rebuilding the body's structure and maintaining overall well-being.

Soothing Stage

The soothing diet serves as a transition phase, both before and after the eliminative diet. It helps individuals gradually shift from the constructive diet to the eliminative diet and vice versa. Additionally, since the digestive system remains at rest during elimination, it requires a gradual reintroduction of foods that demand digestion.

This stage involves consuming easily digestible, soothing foods that help restore digestive function while balancing internal heat generated during elimination. Recommended foods include smoothies, soups, nut milks and porridges.

Eliminative Stage

This phase focuses on detoxification, creating a favourable internal environment free from toxins and accumulated waste. During this stage, fasting is practiced, which may involve consuming only water or a fasting-mimicking diet consisting of very thin juices that provide minimal nutrition and require no digestion.

In my clinic, I refer to these juices as 'coloured water – for example, a small piece of carrot blended in a glass of water. The purpose is primarily psychological, giving individuals a sense of comfort by making them feel that they are not completely deprived. It is crucial to ensure that these juices are not strained, as straining removes fibre, making them as detrimental as refined sugar.

The duration and approach of the eliminative phase vary from person to person and are determined based on their physical, psychological and pathological conditions.

By following these three stages, the naturopathic diet supports detoxification, healing and long-term health restoration, ensuring that the body functions optimally in harmony with nature. As this therapeutic diet requires clinical supervision, which should be learned through experience, I am not elaborating on it in detail.

CHAPTER 4
The Foundation

Rest: The Profound Nothingness

As naturopaths often say, *the body heals itself when given the chance – and that chance is rest.* In today's era, where information is easily available, most people understand the importance of diet and exercise for maintaining health. However, one crucial aspect is often overlooked: rest. Rest is often misunderstood as simply taking a break from physical activity or sleeping after a long day. But true rest is more than just stopping movement; it is about allowing the body and mind to enter a state of deep recovery.

If diet and exercise are the pillars of health, rest is the foundation that holds everything together. Without proper rest, even the best diet and exercise routine cannot bring true healing. The most familiar form of rest is sleep, which is essential for recovery and repair. But in Naturopathy and Yogic healing, along with sleep, we recognise two additional forms of healing rest: fasting and relaxation techniques.

When used wisely and effectively, these three forms of rest – sleep, fasting and relaxation techniques – become powerful tools in the journey of healing and well-being. It is exciting to explore the fascinating science, time-tested methods and incredible benefits of these practices. Together we will unlock the secrets of deep rest and discover how to harness its power for optimum health and vitality.

Sleep: The Body's Natural Medicine

Imagine if there were a medicine that could heal your body, strengthen your immune system, boost your memory and even protect your heart, all without side effects. This medicine already exists and it's free. It's called sleep.

We often think of sleep as just 'resting' or 'shutting down for the night', but in reality it's an active process where the body repairs itself, clears out toxins and restores balance. It's as essential as food and water. Yet, in today's fast-paced world, sleep is often neglected, leading to a host of health problems. Sleep works as nature's most powerful medicine.

Understanding Sleep: Deep Sleep and Dream Sleep

Sleep consists of different phases, each playing a unique role in maintaining health. These phases repeat multiple times throughout the night, forming a complete sleep cycle that lasts about 90 minutes. Scientists divide sleep into two main types: Non-Rapid Eye Movement (NREM) sleep and Rapid Eye Movement (REM) sleep. These names come from how our eyes behave during these stages.

NREM sleep is Non-Rapid Eye Movement sleep because, during this phase, the eyes do not move rapidly. It has three stages, with the third stage being the deepest and most restorative. This deep sleep is when the body repairs itself, strengthens the immune system and builds energy for the next day. Since this phase is crucial for physical recovery, we can refer to it as 'deep sleep'. REM sleep, on the other hand, is called Rapid Eye Movement sleep because the eyes move quickly beneath the eyelids, even though the body remains mostly still. This stage is when most dreams happen and the brain becomes highly active, almost like when we are awake. REM sleep is important for memory, learning and emotional processing, making it fitting to call it 'dream sleep'. So in simple terms, we can think of NREM as deep sleep, where the body heals, and REM as dream sleep, where the brain processes thoughts and emotions. Both are essential for good health, and the body naturally cycles through them several times each night.

Deep Sleep (NREM) – The Body's Repair Mode

Deep sleep, also known as Non-Rapid Eye Movement (NREM) sleep, is when the body enters a deep state of relaxation and restoration. This phase, especially the third stage of NREM, is vital for physical healing. During this time, the body acts like a skilled repair team, fixing damage, rebuilding tissues and restoring energy for the day ahead.

One key process during deep sleep is the release of growth hormone, which supports muscle repair, tissue regeneration and bone strength. This is why deep sleep is crucial for children's growth and for adults recovering from physical exertion or injury. If you've ever felt sore after a workout but refreshed by morning, it's because your body repaired itself during deep sleep.

Another vital function of deep sleep is to strengthen the immune system. During this phase, the body produces immune cells that fight infection and reduce inflammation. Regular, quality deep sleep helps bolster your defences and increases resistance to illness.

Deep sleep is also when the liver, the body's natural detoxifier, performs its most powerful cleansing. Though it works around the clock, its peak detox activity occurs between 1am and 3am. According to traditional healing systems, this is the liver's prime time for clearing toxins from the blood, breaking down chemicals and processing waste accumulated throughout the day. A sluggish liver can contribute to fatigue, poor digestion, hormonal issues and lowered immunity, so this nightly detox is essential for maintaining balance.

You might have heard of the lymphatic system, which helps remove waste from the body. The brain has its own version called the 'glymphatic system'. During deep sleep, this system becomes highly active, flushing out toxins, including beta-amyloid, a protein linked to Alzheimer's disease. When we don't get enough sleep, these toxins build up, increasing the risk of memory problems and neurodegenerative diseases.

Ever noticed how everything feels foggy after a sleepless night? That's because the brain hasn't had the chance to reset. Sleep is essential for memory consolidation, problem-solving and emotional regulation. It's like hitting the 'save' button on everything we've learned and experienced throughout the day.

Dream Sleep (REM) – The Brain's Emotional Reset

After deep sleep the body transitions into REM sleep, also known as dream sleep. This phase is when the brain becomes highly active, almost like it's awake, while the body remains mostly still. REM sleep is where most vivid dreams occur, and it plays a crucial role in processing emotions, strengthening memory and boosting creativity.

Imagine your brain as a busy office that gathers and sorts information all day. REM sleep is like the shift, where everything gets organised, unnecessary clutter is thrown away and important files are stored for future use. This process helps you make sense of the events of the day, reinforcing useful memories while discarding irrelevant ones.

During REM sleep the brain also acts as a built-in therapist. If you've ever gone to bed feeling upset and woken up feeling better, it's because your brain processed your emotions while you were dreaming. Normally, when we experience fear or stress, our brain releases adrenaline, which acts like a fire alarm. But during REM sleep, the alarm is turned off, allowing us to revisit stressful experiences without feeling overwhelmed. It's like watching a scary movie with the sound muted – the experience is still there, but the emotional intensity is reduced. This helps us heal from emotional pain and move forward without unnecessary fear or anxiety.

REM sleep is also a workshop for creativity and problem-solving. The brain takes different pieces of information and combines them in new ways, often leading to fresh ideas and insights. That's why people sometimes wake up with a sudden solution to a problem or a burst of inspiration. Artists, writers and inventors have often credited dreams with sparking their greatest ideas.

Skipping REM sleep has serious consequences. Without enough REM sleep, the brain struggles to manage emotions, leading to irritability, anxiety and difficulty handling stress. Small problems may feel overwhelming and decision-making becomes harder. Over time, lack of REM sleep can affect memory, focus and even creativity.

Magnesium and Sleep: The Missing Link to Deep Rest

Among the many factors that influence sleep, one of the most overlooked is **magnesium,** a mineral essential for relaxation, nervous system function and stress regulation.

Magnesium is involved in over 300 biochemical reactions in the body, many of which directly affect sleep. It helps regulate neurotransmitters – brain chemicals that influence mood and calmness. A key one is **gamma-aminobutyric acid (GABA)**, which acts as a natural relaxant by reducing brain excitability. When magnesium levels are low, GABA function is compromised, making it harder to unwind and fall asleep. That's why magnesium deficiency is often associated with **insomnia, anxiety and restless sleep**.

Magnesium also supports sleep by aiding **melatonin production** – the hormone that governs the body's internal clock or circadian rhythm. A well-regulated rhythm helps us stay alert during the day and sleepy at night. Without enough magnesium, melatonin levels may drop, disrupting natural sleep-wake cycles.

Another important role of magnesium is in **stress regulation**. The body's stress system, known as the **hypothalamic-pituitary-adrenal (HPA) axis**, controls the release of cortisol. When stress is chronic, cortisol stays elevated, making it harder to relax. Magnesium helps modulate this process, keeping cortisol in check and helping the body shift into a restful state.

Finally, magnesium is crucial for **muscle relaxation**. It balances calcium levels in muscle cells, preventing them from staying in a contracted state. When magnesium is lacking, muscles may remain tense, leading to cramps, spasms or **restless legs syndrome**, all of which can disrupt sleep.

Dreams: A Sign You're Getting Good Sleep

A lot of people think dreaming means their sleep is disturbed, but it's actually the opposite – dreaming is a sign that you're getting enough deep sleep! During REM sleep (the phase when most dreams happen) your body's stress hormones, especially cortisol, drop to their lowest levels. This helps your mind reset and recover from daily stress. Dreams also help you process emotions in a safe way, kind of like your brain's built-in therapy. Plus, with stress hormones at their lowest, your brain gets creative, making connections and coming up with new ideas. So if you're dreaming, it's a good thing; it means your sleep is doing its job, helping you wake up feeling refreshed and balanced!

Sleep and the Immune System: Your Body's Defence Mechanism

Ever noticed how all you want to do is sleep when you're sick? That's not laziness, it's your body's natural defence system in action. Sleep is one of the most powerful ways your body fights off infections. While you rest, your immune system ramps up, producing **cytokines** – proteins that help respond to infection, inflammation and stress.

But when sleep is lacking, your immune system suffers. Studies show that sleep-deprived people are more prone to colds, flu and other infections. It's not just about feeling tired; poor sleep weakens immune defences and increases inflammation, contributing to long-term health issues like **heart disease, diabetes** and even **cancer**.

One critical immune component influenced by sleep is the **Natural Killer Cells (NKCs)** – the immune system's sharpshooters, trained to eliminate virus-infected and cancerous cells. Without enough sleep, these NKCs are pulled off duty. Research reveals that sleeping less than six hours can reduce NKC activity by up to **70 percent**, leaving your body vulnerable.

Think of a sleepless night as lowering your defences and giving pathogens a free pass. On the other hand, sleeping seven to nine hours each night keeps NKCs functioning well and inflammation under control.

Sleep also balances **stress hormones** like cortisol. When you're not well-rested, cortisol stays high and further suppresses NKCs. The deepest stages of sleep, especially **non-REM (NREM)** sleep, are essential for restoring NKC activity. Your **circadian rhythm** – the body's internal clock – relies on regular, quality sleep to regulate immune cells and function effectively. So the next time you consider sacrificing sleep for work or entertainment, remember, it's not just about energy, it's about keeping your internal defence system strong.

During deep sleep, your body boosts insulin sensitivity and supports glucose uptake. Skipping sleep disrupts this process, throwing blood sugar levels off and raising the risk of insulin resistance and type 2 diabetes. Research confirms that sleep-deprived individuals often struggle with glucose regulation and fat storage, and are more prone to obesity and metabolic syndrome.

A recent study found that people who identify as 'night owls' have a 46 percent higher risk of developing type 2 diabetes than those with more neutral sleep patterns, even after adjusting for age, weight, lifestyle and diet. Researchers believe this is due to circadian misalignment – when your internal clock is out of sync with societal routines, causing metabolic disruptions.

Ever crave junk food after a poor night's sleep? That's because sleep loss messes with your hunger hormones – **ghrelin** (which makes you hungry) increases, while **leptin** (which signals fullness) decreases. This makes you hungrier and more likely to overeat, increasing the risk of weight gain.

Poor sleep doesn't just affect appetite. It also impacts how the body processes and stores fat. People who consistently sleep less than six hours often see higher BMI, even with a healthy diet and regular exercise. This is mainly due to hormonal imbalances. Low leptin and high ghrelin levels stimulate cravings for high-calorie, sugary and processed foods.

Sleep and Memory: How Sleep Turns Experiences into Learning

Think of your brain as a library, and your daily experiences as books piled up on a table in the hippocampus – the brain's temporary storage bin. Throughout the day, you gather new information, but unless it's properly organised it won't be very useful.

When you sleep, your brain acts like a librarian, carefully sorting these books and placing them in the right sections of your 'memory library' – different parts of the brain responsible for emotions, movement, knowledge and problem-solving. But memory is more than just storage; to truly learn, the brain needs to connect new experiences with old ones, creating a deeper understanding of the world.

During deep sleep, the brain works like a builder, strengthening important memories by moving them from the hippocampus, where they are temporarily stored, to the neocortex, where they become part of long-term memory. This process ensures that the information you gather during the day is retained for the future. Meanwhile, REM sleep, the stage in which we dream, acts like a networker, linking new memories with past experiences. This helps us recognise patterns, make better decisions and even enhance creativity.

For example, an adult knows not to eat spoiled food because they have learned from experience that it can make them sick. A child, however, may not avoid it unless they have already experienced food poisoning. These connections – linking past experiences to new situations – happen while we sleep. Without good sleep, the 'shelves' of our memory become unstable, making it harder to learn, recall information or think clearly.

The Leptin-Ghrelin Mechanism

The **Leptin-Ghrelin Mechanism** is like a built-in food regulator in your body, but sometimes it can go haywire.

Ghrelin is the little troublemaker that makes your stomach growl, literally. Think of it as 'Ghrelin the Greedy', always whispering (or sometimes shouting) *"Grrrr… I'm hungry!"* the moment your stomach starts feeling empty. It's made in the stomach and tells your brain to eat. Normally, once you eat, ghrelin calms down, and Leptin – the 'I'm full' signal – steps in to say, *"Alright, we're good, stop eating."* Leptin is released by fat cells and keeps your appetite in check.

But here's where things go wrong. When you overeat frequently, especially processed foods and sugars, your brain starts ignoring leptin's signals. This is called leptin resistance, and it's a vicious cycle. Since your brain isn't recognising that you're full, you keep eating, which leads to more fat storage. More fat should mean more leptin, but because your brain is now numb to it, you never feel satisfied. Meanwhile, ghrelin stays loud, constantly convincing you that you need more food. This cycle makes weight management tough, because the natural hunger and fullness signals are all out of sync.

To break this cycle, the key is restoring leptin sensitivity and keeping ghrelin under control. Prioritising good sleep, eating whole, unprocessed foods, managing stress and staying physically active help rebalance these hormones. When leptin and ghrelin work as they should, your hunger cues start making sense again and you regain control over your appetite.

What we think about just before sleep also plays a significant role in memory and emotional processing. The thoughts, emotions and images we focus on before drifting off can influence what the brain prioritises during the night. If we go to sleep with stress, worry or negative emotions, the brain may reinforce those patterns, leading to restless sleep and heightened anxiety the next day. On the other hand, reflecting on positive thoughts, gratitude or learning experiences can help strengthen useful memories, improve problem-solving and promote emotional well-being. This is why practices like reading something uplifting, visualising goals or meditating before sleep can shape not only our dreams, but also our waking mind-set.

The Importance of a Full Sleep Cycle

A complete sleep cycle lasts about 90 minutes, and we go through four to six cycles per night. However, not all sleep is equal. If sleep is interrupted frequently, the body may not complete all the necessary stages, leading to tiredness even after a long night in bed.

The amount of sleep needed varies by age:

- Adults - 7–9 hours per night.
- Teenagers - 8–10 hours to support growth and brain development.
- Children - 9–12 hours to fuel their rapid physical and mental development.

If you wake up feeling tired despite sleeping for long hours, it may not be about how much sleep you get, but how well you cycle through deep sleep and dream sleep. Poor sleep quality can affect mood, memory and overall health.

Ever wonder if sleeping six hours at night and taking a two-hour nap during the day is just as good as a full eight hours of sleep? It might seem like it adds up, but your body doesn't work that way. Sleep follows a natural cycle – deep sleep happens mostly in the early night, when your body repairs itself and clears out toxins, while dream sleep (REM) comes later, helping you process emotions and memories. When sleep is broken, you miss out on these critical phases, leaving you feeling groggy, tired and out of sync. A nap might give you a quick boost, but it can't fully replace deep, uninterrupted sleep at night.

Sleep Isn't Optional – It's Mandatory!

The science is clear: sleep isn't just a break from daily life; it's a biological necessity. Skipping sleep doesn't just make you groggy – it can lead to serious long-term health consequences. Sleep affects everything from your heart and metabolism to your weight and brain function.

Instead of treating sleep as something we can sacrifice, we should start seeing it as the foundation of good health, if diet and exercise are the pillars. Prioritising sleep hygiene can go a long way in preventing chronic diseases and improving overall well-being.

So the next time you think about skipping sleep, remember: Your body and mind are counting on you to rest. Give yourself the sleep you deserve!

How to Improve Your Sleep Quality

The good news is, you don't need to make drastic changes to sleep better. Small, mindful adjustments can make a big difference in improving sleep quality and overall well-being.

- **Respect Your Sleep** – Don't take sleep lightly. Recognise its importance and give it the priority it deserves.
- **Stick to a Consistent Schedule** – Going to bed and waking up at the same time every day helps regulate your body's internal clock, making it easier to fall asleep and wake up refreshed.
- **Create a Sleep-Friendly Environment** – A cool, dark and quiet room sends the right signals to your body that it's time to rest.
- **Limit Screen Time Before Bed** – The blue light from screens interferes with melatonin, the hormone that helps you sleep. Try to switch off devices at least an hour before bedtime.
- **Practice Relaxation Techniques** – Activities like meditation, deep breathing or journaling can calm the mind and prepare you for restful sleep.

- **Watch What You Consume** – Avoid caffeine, heavy meals and stimulants close to bedtime, as they can disrupt your sleep cycle.
- **Get Plenty of Natural Light** – Exposure to sunlight during the day helps regulate your circadian rhythm, making it easier to fall asleep at night.

By making these small, consistent changes, you can improve your sleep quality and wake up feeling more energised, focussed and ready for the day ahead.

Early to Bed, Early to Rise – Does It Work for Everyone?

We often hear that waking up early is the key to health and success, but in reality, sleep patterns aren't the same for everyone. Biologically and evolutionarily, humans are designed to live in tribes, where some people naturally sleep early while others stay awake later. This way, there's always someone alert, reducing the chances of being caught off guard by predators. So, your sleep pattern should align with what feels natural to *your* body rather than forcing an unnatural schedule.

That said, one universal truth is that the body goes through essential repair processes between 11pm and 3am, particularly for hormone regulation, immune function and cellular recovery. No matter your sleep preference, it's important to be in deep sleep during this window for optimal health. The key is to find a sleep schedule that suits your natural rhythm while ensuring you get quality, restorative sleep!

Fasting: The Supreme Remedy

The Story of a Wonder Drug – and the Ancient Secret Within You

Many years ago, on the mysterious and faraway Easter Island – known to locals as Rapa Nui – scientists digging through the soil made a surprising discovery. Hidden in the earth was a special kind of bacteria that produced a substance later named **rapamycin**. At first it seemed like just another antifungal agent, but as researchers studied it more deeply, they uncovered something remarkable: rapamycin could slow down aging, fight cancer and even extend life in animals. How? By switching off a powerful growth signal in our cells called **mTOR,** a master controller of how fast cells grow, divide and age. When mTOR is turned down, the body focusses less on growth and more on healing, repair and regeneration. However Rapamycin, being a drug, comes with its own side effects, like immunosuppression.

But here's the real twist in the story: What rapamycin does in the lab, your body already knows how to do on its own. You don't need to travel to a distant island or take a special pill. You simply need to bring a pause to eating - Practice Fasting.. When you stop eating for a period – whether it's skipping a meal, practicing intermittent fasting or following a guided therapeutic fast – your body naturally lowers mTOR activity. It enters a state of deep healing, clearing out old, damaged cells and renewing itself from within. This is exactly what Naturopathy has taught for centuries. In naturopathic medicine, therapeutic fasting is not just about skipping meals; it's a structured, safe and deeply cleansing process that allows the body to reset and rejuvenate. In essence, fasting is your body's own version of rapamycin – free, natural and profoundly healing – rooted in ancient wisdom and now confirmed by modern science.

For those who haven't yet come across this beautiful yet powerful healing method of fasting, get ready to learn something truly amazing. This is going to be one of the most enlightening parts of the journey we've been traveling so far!

Some of you might be wondering why fasting is included here under the topic of rest. After all, fasting is about eating… or rather, not eating, right? Shouldn't it be discussed under Diet? In Naturopathy, we say '*Langhanam Paramaushadham*' – which means pause or break is the supreme remedy. Fasting is the most effective way to give the body the deep rest it truly needs.

Dr Babu Joseph, former Director of the National Institute of Naturopathy, Pune, who unravelled the beautiful science of naturopathic healing for me, explains fasting in the simplest yet most profound way:

"Fasting is complete rest – physical, mental, sensory, emotional and social (I often include social media in my talks). It involves total, voluntary abstinence from anything that requires digestion or provides external energy, except water, for a specific purpose and period of time."

Fasting is not depriving the body of something; rather, it is a gift, an opportunity for the body to activate its natural self-healing mechanisms. When the body is freed from the constant task of digestion, it redirects energy toward repair, detoxification and renewal. This state of inner cleansing strengthens immunity, balances metabolism and promotes overall well-being.

By deciding to undergo fasting, we reclaim our power, along with all the magical therapeutic benefits it possesses. Food being the greatest addiction, we have become so powerless in saying no to food that it has become the root of most health issues we humans suffer from today. By undergoing fasting, we take back control from one of the strongest compulsions we have, allowing our body to reset, our mind to refocus and our spirit to reconnect with balance.

By understanding fasting as the ultimate form of rest, we begin to see its profound impact on our health. But how exactly does it work at a deeper level? Let's explore to uncover the incredible ways fasting transforms our body at the cellular level.

Unlocking the Power of Fasting: The Science, Benefits and Cellular Mechanisms

How Does Fasting Work at the Cellular Level?

Throughout our lives, we eat regularly, often much more than our body actually requires. But have you ever wondered why our body tends to store excess energy? The answer lies in our genes, which carry the memories of countless generations before us. Our ancestors, from hunter-gatherers to early civilisations, endured periods of famine and scarcity. To survive, their bodies evolved a mechanism to store excess food as fat, preparing for times when food might not be available.

Even though modern life rarely presents the same survival challenges, our genes still operate with the ancient fear of starvation. So when we overeat, our body sees it as an opportunity to stockpile energy, even though the anticipated famine never arrives. As a result, excess energy accumulates, leading to long-term imbalances in health.

But what happens when we fast? When we voluntarily pause food intake, as guided by naturopathic principles, we interrupt this cycle of constant consumption and storage. After about 12 hours of fasting, the body shifts gears; it begins breaking down stored fat for energy instead of relying on glucose (sugar) from food.

And this is just the beginning! If we extend fasting beyond 12 hours to 14, 16, 24 or even 36 hours or more, the body activates one of its most fascinating self-repair mechanisms: **Autophagy,** by the inhibition of mTOR, a cellular mechanism I mentioned earlier. This process allows cells to recycle damaged components, remove toxins and enhance overall cellular function, unlocking extraordinary health benefits.

Unveiling Autophagy: The Body's Silent Rebirth

Imagine waking up one day to find that your neighbourhood has been placed under a sudden containment lockdown due to an outbreak of a rapidly spreading infection. You're confined to your home, unable to go out or get anything from outside. Hours pass and hunger starts creeping in. You head to the kitchen, only to realise that your stock of groceries and fresh vegetables has run out.

What Would You Do?

You'd likely start searching for leftovers in the pantry, scavenging through the refrigerator for anything usable. You might even get creative, recycling, repurposing and making the most of what's available to sustain yourself.

Now here's the amazing part – your body does the exact same thing when you fast! When you stop eating for an extended period, your body can't rely on fresh energy from food. So it switches to survival mode and starts looking for 'leftovers' inside you – old, damaged or unnecessary parts of cells. Instead of letting these waste materials build up, your body recycles and repurposes them into new, useful components.

Body's Adaptive Response to Fasting

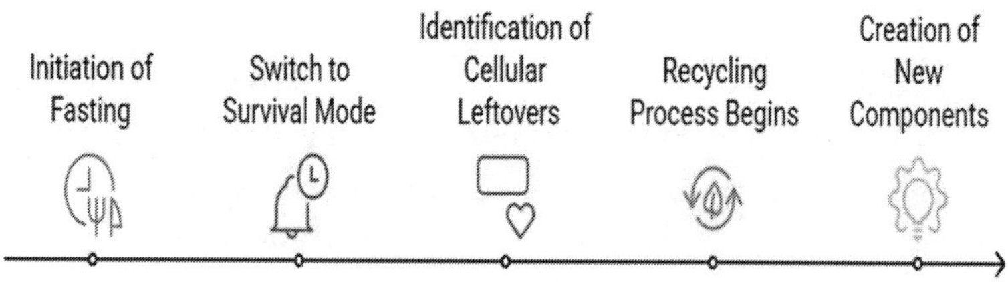

This natural cleaning process is called Autophagy, derived from Greek, which literally means 'self-eating'. It's like a deep cleanse for your cells!

Autophagy is a highly regulated biological process that activates when the body has depleted its immediate energy reserves and shifts into a state of metabolic adaptation. Just like searching for food in your pantry, your cells begin scavenging for old, misfolded or damaged proteins to repurpose.

- Aged or damaged cell components that no longer function efficiently are broken down and recycled.
- Accumulated proteins (which contribute to neurodegenerative diseases like Alzheimer's) are cleared out.

- Old energy factories in the cell (mitochondria) are removed to make way for fresh, more efficient ones.
- Even harmful invaders, like viruses hiding in cells, can be destroyed.

Through autophagy, these unnecessary components are broken down and either used for energy or replaced with fresh, functional ones, allowing the body to cleanse itself at a deep cellular level.

This process doesn't just prevent disease; it's a key mechanism for longevity, metabolic health and cellular rejuvenation. Research has shown that fasting-induced autophagy can reduce inflammation, improve brain function and support healthy aging.

But here's the thing – autophagy doesn't start right away. It needs time. Studies suggest that it begins to increase significantly after about 16–24 hours of fasting and works even better with longer fasts.

I have provided a simplified explanation of a highly intricate biochemical process, but at its core, autophagy is the body's way of protecting, rejuvenating and optimising itself, triggered by fasting. So when you fast, you're not just skipping meals, you're giving your body a chance to renew, heal and perform its own deep cleaning.

Unlocking Profound Health Benefits

While we have already explored the concept of **autophagy,** or the process by which cells clean and repair themselves, it is only one part of the broader picture. The health benefits of fasting extend far beyond cellular renewal. They reach into nearly every system of the body, enhancing metabolism, brain function, cardiovascular health and even longevity.

Understanding these mechanisms can transform the way we perceive fasting – not as deprivation, but as an intentional and scientifically backed practice that optimises well-being. Let's explore how fasting actively contributes to a healthier, more resilient body.

1. Brain Health and Cognitive Function: Sharpening the Mind

Fasting does more than cleanse the body; it strengthens the brain. When we fast, the brain increases production of brain-derived neurotrophic factor (BDNF), a protein vital for the growth, protection and survival of neurons. Higher BDNF levels are linked to better learning, sharper memory and improved mental clarity (Mattson et al., 2018).

Fasting also boosts the brain's energy efficiency by shifting from glucose to ketone metabolism. Ketones are energy molecules made by the liver when the body burns fat, usually during fasting, low-carb diets or intense exercise. They offer a more stable, efficient fuel for both brain and muscles, providing neuroprotective effects and potentially lowering the risk of conditions like Alzheimer's and Parkinson's (Cunnane et al., 2016).

In addition to fuelling the brain with ketones, fasting lowers inflammation and enhances neural plasticity, our brain's ability to adapt, form new pathways and strengthen old ones. Reduced inflammation helps protect brain cells, while improved plasticity boosts learning, memory and overall cognitive function. Together, these benefits foster clearer thinking, sharper focus and long-term brain health.

2. Fat Loss and Metabolic Flexibility: Teaching the Body to Burn Fat

Beyond fat loss, fasting enhances metabolic flexibility, the body's ability to seamlessly switch between fuel sources. This means that over time, people who incorporate fasting into their lifestyle become more efficient at using stored fat for energy, reducing dependency on constant food intake.

Moreover, fasting regulates hunger hormones like ghrelin and leptin, leading to better appetite control and reduced cravings (Flanagan et al., 2020). Instead of feeling controlled by hunger, fasting teaches the body how to sustain energy levels without frequent eating.

3. Insulin Sensitivity and Blood Sugar Regulation: Optimising Metabolic Health

Fasting has a profound impact on insulin sensitivity, which is the body's ability to use insulin effectively. When insulin sensitivity is high, cells can easily absorb glucose from the bloodstream, preventing excessive blood sugar spikes (Patterson & Sears, 2017).

However, when insulin sensitivity declines, insulin resistance sets in, which leads to metabolic disorders such as type 2 diabetes, obesity and heart disease. Studies have shown that intermittent fasting significantly lowers fasting blood sugar and insulin levels, allowing the body to reset its glucose metabolism (Anton et al., 2018).

By giving the digestive system a break, fasting allows insulin levels to drop, enhancing the body's ability to efficiently process and store energy. This makes it a powerful tool in both preventing and managing metabolic disorders.

4. Inflammation Reduction: Cooling the Fire Within

Fasting helps counteract inflammation by reducing levels of pro-inflammatory cytokines – molecules that signal the immune system to trigger an inflammatory response (Moro et al., 2016).

Moreover, fasting initiates a process where damaged or dysfunctional immune cells are removed and replaced with new, healthier cells. This means that rather than merely suppressing inflammation, fasting actively rejuvenates the immune system, making the body more resilient against infections and diseases (Cheng et al., 2014).

5. Cardiovascular Health: Strengthening the Heart

Heart disease remains one of the leading causes of death worldwide, but fasting offers a natural way to protect and strengthen the cardiovascular system. It does this in several ways:

- Lowers LDL Cholesterol and Triglycerides: Fasting reduces harmful cholesterol levels, which are major contributors to heart disease (Tinsley & La Bounty, 2015).
- Increases HDL ('good') Cholesterol: This helps maintain a healthy balance of fats in the blood (Harvie & Howell, 2017).
- Reduces Blood Pressure: Fasting improves vascular function by increasing nitric oxide production, which helps dilate blood vessels and enhance circulation (Wilhelmi de Toledo et al., 2019).
- Lowers Oxidative Stress: By reducing free radicals, fasting protects blood vessels from damage and premature aging (Longo & Mattson, 2014).

The cumulative effect is a stronger heart, healthier arteries and a reduced risk of cardiovascular disease, all without the need for medications or extreme lifestyle interventions.

6. Longevity and Healing: A Blueprint for a Longer, Healthier Life

One of the most exciting discoveries in fasting research is its ability to activate genes associated with longevity and stress resistance. When the body experiences mild stress from fasting, it triggers adaptive responses that increase lifespan, enhance repair mechanisms and reduce the likelihood of age-related diseases (Brandhorst et al., 2015).

Fasting stimulates the production of **sirtuins**, proteins that regulate ageing, DNA repair and cellular protection. Studies on animals and humans suggest that fasting extends life expectancy by slowing down cellular ageing and reducing the risk of chronic diseases (Madeo et al., 2019).

In short, by fasting regularly, we give our bodies the tools they need to heal, renew and ultimately thrive for years to come.

Incorporating Fasting into Your Lifestyle: A Practical Approach to Sustainable Health

Fasting is not just a theory; it's a time-tested practice backed by science and centuries of traditional wisdom. The real question isn't *"Does fasting work?"* but rather, *"How can I make fasting a natural part of my life?"*

The beauty of fasting is that it's flexible. It doesn't have to be extreme or difficult, and you don't need to starve yourself to experience its benefits. Whether through intermittent fasting, extended fasting or time-restricted eating, anyone can integrate fasting into their daily routine in a way that suits their body, lifestyle and health goals.

But here's the key: fasting should be tailored to you. Your body type, habits, energy levels and overall health should guide how to do the fasting. A great way to start is by having an early dinner and a late breakfast, a practice we call **Brunch** in Naturopathy. This simple adjustment naturally creates a 14-hour gap between two meals, giving your body time to rest, digest and begin the healing process.

Once you're comfortable with this, you can gradually explore deeper fasting:

- 24-hour fasting – From dinner to the next day's dinner, giving your digestive system a full reset.
- 36-hour fasting – Two nights and one full day without food, allowing deeper detoxification and healing.

Doing this once a week or once every two weeks can be highly beneficial. But beyond this, it's always best to fast under the guidance of a qualified naturopathy physician in a healing retreat or in-patient setup.

Fasting for Healing: The Right Way to Do It

If you're someone who has never skipped a meal, fasting won't be easy at first. Your body will resist. You might experience hunger cravings, abdominal discomfort, headaches or fatigue – this is what we call the 'welcome to detox' message. These are normal and temporary, and they often pass as your body adjusts. But if you're new to fasting, having a Naturopathy doctor's support can help you push through these initial challenges safely.

There's no doubt that fasting promotes healing. However, if you have a medical condition, discomfort or are on medication, it is important to always consult a healthcare expert before fasting. Naturopathy follows a fundamental principle:

> "The food you eat while diseased does not nourish the body – it feeds the disease."

This highlights why fasting is especially important during illness. However, therapeutic fasting must always be done under medical supervision.

Golden Rules for Safe and Effective Therapeutic Fasting

If you want to experience the true power of fasting, follow these key principles:

- Never practice dry fasting. Always drink enough water – water is your detox agent during fasting.
- Avoid extreme physical or mental exertion. For instance, if you're fasting while engaging in a heated argument, you're not really fasting – you're just fighting!
- Ease into fasting gradually. Don't rush into it aggressively. Follow the Naturopathy diet pattern, which includes a constructive phase, a soothing phase and an eliminative phase, to prepare your body for fasting.
- Fast with a positive mindset. You're not depriving yourself; you're doing this voluntarily, and you are in control.
- Don't use fasting as a weight-loss trick. Fasting is for detoxification, repair and healing. While you may lose weight during fasting, it's temporary. Fasting is about health, not just shedding pounds.

- Break your fast wisely. Naturopaths say, "Any fool can fast, but only a wise person knows how to break a fast properly." After fasting, avoid jumping straight into heavy, spicy or processed foods. Reintroduce food slowly and gently.

As you begin your fasting journey, remind yourself that every moment spent in fasting is a moment spent in healing. You are giving your body the chance to repair, reset and thrive. So embrace it, not as a struggle, but as a powerful tool for lifelong health.

How to Practice and Break Fasting Safely

Fasting has many benefits, and just as important as fasting itself is knowing how to break it wisely. After a fast, your body needs nourishing, wholesome foods to rebuild and recover.

A common misconception is that feeling tired during a fast means your body is out of energy and it's time to eat. But let's view it differently. Picture a lion that hasn't eaten for days. If fasting made it weak, it couldn't hunt. But instead, it becomes sharper and more focussed, ready to chase its prey. Our bodies work in much the same way. Fasting doesn't sap energy; it enhances it, helping us stay alert and responsive.

When food isn't available, the body doesn't shut down, it adapts. It switches to a more efficient energy system. If fasting truly left us weak, our ancestors wouldn't have survived. They needed to stay sharp to search for food. During fasting, the body increases hormones like norepinephrine, which enhance alertness and metabolism. In fact, research shows short-term fasting can boost metabolic rate by up to 14 percent, helping the body use energy more efficiently.

Still, it's important to know when to break a fast. Not every hunger pang means the body is in distress. True signals include persistent hunger, dizziness, weakness or mental confusion. If you're shaking, extremely hungry or losing muscle, it's time to eat. But a bit of tiredness or food cravings alone don't necessarily mean the fast should end – these often pass as your body adjusts.

Fasting should energise you, not drain you. If someone feels constantly fatigued while fasting, they might need more water or electrolytes, or a different approach. When done properly, fasting clears the mind, strengthens the body and taps into the natural resilience built into us, just like that lion, primed for the hunt.

To fast effectively and practice it therapeutically, you need clarity on two key concepts:

1. Fasting is not starvation.
2. Hunger is not appetite. (already discussed under Diet)

Fasting vs Starvation: Understanding the Difference

In 2007, as part of our initiative to popularise Naturopathy & Yoga among the general public, the Indian Naturopathy & Yoga Graduates Medical Association (INYGMA) in Kerala decided to undertake a seven-day fasting event in Thiruvananthapuram, the capital of the state. The purpose was to create awareness about the benefits of fasting and natural healing while demonstrating the principles we advocate.

As part of this campaign, a group of Naturopathy doctors, including myself, decided to visit the then Home Minister and Chief Minister of Kerala to personally invite them to the event. When we met the Home Minister, he listened to our plans with great concern. With genuine sincerity, he said, "Are you all starving for seven days? If you have any demands, we can consider them. There is no need to go to such an extreme." His reaction reflected the common misunderstanding many people have about fasting, equating it with starvation rather than a purposeful and controlled practice for health and well-being.

Later, we visited the Chief Minister, a person well aware of Naturopathy and someone who had personally undergone naturopathic treatments in his life. His response was completely different. With a warm smile, he said, "A seven-day fast? Very good! It will make all of you healthier. My best wishes!" His words reflected an understanding of the true essence of fasting, not as deprivation but as a practice of healing and rejuvenation.

I narrated this story, because it beautifully highlights how fasting is often misunderstood by those unfamiliar with its principles, while those who have experienced it first-hand recognise its immense benefits. It reinforced our belief in the need to educate more people about Naturopathy, fasting and the body's natural ability to heal when given the right conditions.

At first glance, fasting and starvation may seem similar; they both involve going without food. But they differ significantly in purpose, effect and impact. The key distinction is that fasting is a choice, while starvation is a crisis.

Fasting is a voluntary practice, done for health, spiritual or therapeutic reasons. Starvation, however, is an involuntary lack of food, often due to poverty, illness or scarcity. While fasting is controlled and temporary, starvation is prolonged and life-threatening. During starvation, the body enters a desperate state, breaking down not just fat, but also muscle and organs to survive.

A key difference lies in control and duration. Fasting is time-bound – 16 hours, a day or a few days – allowing the body to tap into beneficial metabolic states. Starvation extends beyond that, causing the body to burn through all reserves, including vital tissues, which can lead to severe damage or death.

The body responds differently to each. In fasting, the body adapts by increasing hormones that boost alertness and metabolism. In starvation, once fat stores are gone, the body breaks down muscles and organs, leading to malnutrition, weakened immunity and eventual failure of vital systems.

There's also a mental difference. Fasting, while challenging, often brings clarity, focus and a sense of renewal. It can feel empowering and purposeful. Starvation is traumatic, marked by constant hunger, anxiety and mental fog. It causes deep emotional and physical suffering, with dangerous long-term consequences.

Starvation is not a choice – it leads to nutrient depletion, extreme weakness and serious complications. Unlike the structured and beneficial nature of fasting, starvation requires urgent intervention to prevent irreversible harm.

During fasting, it's crucial to know that **Hunger Is Not the Same As Appetite**. In the early stages, hunger pangs may appear as your body adapts. But these typically fade once fat burning begins. This is a natural shift in metabolism, not an emergency.

Understanding the difference between hunger and appetite is one of fasting's greatest lessons. Hunger is your body's real call for fuel; appetite is often a passing urge. By tuning into your body, you develop a healthier relationship with food and make fasting more empowering.

Relaxation: The Art of Alert-ful and Restorative Rest

We often use the word rest and relaxation as synonyms, but it is not the same. The art of relaxation is not simply the absence of effort, but a conscious state of being where both the body and mind are at ease, yet alert.

Relaxation is an intentional process of unwinding the nervous system, bringing the body into balance and allowing the mind to reset while maintaining awareness. It is not just about lying down or closing one's eyes, but about cultivating a state where stress is released, energy is restored and clarity emerges.

In the tradition of Yoga & Naturopathy, relaxation is considered an essential practice for health. Yogic relaxation techniques have been practiced for centuries to harmonise the body's physiological functions and calm the fluctuations of the mind. These practices go beyond temporary relief from stress; they work at a deep level to reset the nervous system, improve circulation and enhance mental focus. Scientific research now validates what ancient traditions have known for millennia: Structured relaxation techniques can significantly lower cortisol levels, reduce inflammation, improve heart rate variability and boost overall well-being.

One of the fundamental relaxation techniques in Yoga is *Shavasana*, or the Corpse Pose. Despite its simplicity, it is one of the most powerful ways to bring the body into a deeply restorative state. When practiced correctly, it allows for a full-body release of tension, facilitating deep nervous system relaxation. Other techniques include *Yoga Nidra*, a guided relaxation method that induces a state of conscious sleep, where the body rests deeply while the mind remains aware, and *Pranayama*, or breath work, which helps regulate the autonomic nervous system and bring about a profound sense of calm.

Relaxation techniques can be categorised based on their depth and purpose:

- Deep Relaxation Technique (DRT): This method takes the body into a state of profound rest, often practiced at the end of a yoga session. It involves progressive relaxation of different body parts and is highly effective in reducing chronic stress and fatigue.
- Quick Relaxation Technique (QRT): A shorter version of deep relaxation, this practice is designed to bring immediate relief from stress and tension in just a few minutes. It involves mindful breathing and gentle body awareness, making it ideal for use during breaks in a busy day.
- Instant Relaxation Technique (IRT): As the name suggests, this is a rapid method to calm the body and mind within seconds. Often used before important tasks or stressful situations, it typically involves a deep inhalation, full-body stretch and a quick release of tension through an exhalation.

The benefits of relaxation are immense. When we truly relax, the body shifts from a state of stress-driven survival to one of healing and rejuvenation. Muscle tension dissolves, breathing becomes deeper and more rhythmic, digestion improves and the immune system strengthens. Mental clarity increases as the mind becomes free from excessive chatter. Emotionally, relaxation creates a space for self-awareness, helping us manage emotions more effectively and respond to life with greater ease.

In today's fast-paced world, relaxation is no longer a luxury, but a necessity. Learning how to enter a state of deep relaxation consciously, without external stimulants like television, social media or sedatives, is an art that can transform health and well-being. By making relaxation a daily practice, we cultivate resilience, enhance our ability to handle stress and allow the body to function at its optimal capacity.

Relaxation is not about doing nothing; it is about doing something powerful. It is an active surrender, a conscious letting go, a gateway to profound healing. Through the art of relaxation we unlock a deeper dimension of rest, one that restores not just the body, but also the mind and soul.

References:

1. Anton, S. D., et al. (2018). "Flipping the Metabolic Switch: Understanding and Applying the Health Benefits of Fasting." *Obesity*, 26(2), 254-268.
2. Brandhorst, S., et al. (2015). "Fasting-mimicking diet and markers/risk factors for aging, diabetes, cancer, and cardiovascular disease." *Cell Metabolism*, 22(2), 86-99.
3. Cheng, C. W., et al. (2014). "Prolonged fasting reduces IGF-1/PKA to promote hematopoietic-stem-cell-based regeneration and reverse immunosuppression." *Cell Stem Cell*, 14(6), 810-823.
4. Longo, V. D., & Mattson, M. P. (2014). "Fasting: Molecular Mechanisms and Clinical Applications." *Cell Metabolism*, 19(2), 181-192.
5. Madeo, F., et al. (2019). "Fasting-Mimicking Diets for Longevity." *Cell Metabolism*, 30(2), 126-140.
6. Mattson, M. P., et al. (2018). "Intermittent metabolic switching, neuroplasticity, and brain health." *Nature Reviews Neuroscience*, 19(2), 63-80.

CHAPTER 5

The Essential

Activity - We Are Not Born as Trees

"Inactivity is death. Activity is life."

- Swami Vivekananda

Why Do We Need to Move?

Have you ever wondered why we need to exercise? After all, no other animal goes to the gym! From an evolutionary and biological perspective, if we were still living as hunter-gatherers climbing trees for fruits, chasing rabbits for food or sprinting away from predators, we wouldn't need structured workouts. Movement would be built into our survival.

But today? Food comes straight to our table, transportation is effortless and comfort is the new normal. Unfortunately, our bodies haven't adapted to this sedentary lifestyle. We are designed for movement – our muscles, bones and joints are built to squat, walk, run, jump, climb and swim. The less we move, the more we lose.

If we ignore this fundamental need for movement, our bodies start deteriorating. And science backs this up with some hard facts.

What Happens When We Stop Moving? - here are the facts and figures:

We lose flexibility: Our joints and muscles stiffen with age, losing 6–10 percent of flexibility every decade after 30 [1]. That's why stretching and mobility exercises become so important.

- Our muscles shrink: We lose 3–8 percent of muscle mass per decade after 30. If we don't do strength training, this rate accelerates to

15 percent per decade after 60! Less muscle means weaker bones, lower metabolism and higher risk of injury [2].

- Our heart and lungs weaken: Our ability to use oxygen declines by 10 percent per decade after 30. If we stay active, this loss reduces to just 5 percent per decade, but if we stay sedentary, it's much worse [3].
- We increase our risk of an early death: Studies show that people who don't exercise regularly have a 30–50 percent higher risk of premature death compared to those who stay active [4]. Just 150 minutes of moderate exercise per week can cut the risk of dying early by 30–35 percent [4].
- We lose grip strength, an indicator of aging: After 40, our grip strength declines by 1–2 percent per year. Why does this matter? Studies link grip strength to overall health and longevity. Weak grip = weak body = higher risk of falls and fractures [5].
- Falls become deadly: The leading cause of injury-related deaths in adults over 65 is falling. This happens because of muscle loss, balance issues and weak bones [5].
- Our brain health declines: Regular exercise reduces the risk of dementia and Alzheimer's by 30–40 percent! Movement isn't just for our body – it's critical for our brain [6].
- We shorten our lifespan: Active people live 3-6 years longer on average. Even as little as 10 minutes of movement a day lowers the risk of early death by 10 percent [7].
- Walking 7,000 steps per day has been linked to a 25 percent lower risk of depression. Additionally, for every extra 1,000 steps taken – up to 10,000 steps daily – the likelihood of experiencing depressive episodes decreases by about 9 percent.

The Solution? Move like our Ancestors!

The answer to staying strong, flexible and mobile is in moving the way our ancestors did. Human bodies are designed for natural, functional movements that keep us fit, agile and resilient. Squatting wasn't an exercise; it was a natural resting position that maintained hip mobility and supported digestion. Walking was the default mode of transportation, ensuring endurance and cardiovascular health. Running wasn't just sport – it was essential for survival, whether chasing prey or escaping predators. Jumping developed agility, coordination and explosive strength. Swimming built endurance and provided a full-body workout that was easy on the joints. Climbing, an ability we share with our ape relatives, engages the entire body, strengthening muscles and improving grip strength. These are the movements our bodies evolved to perform, and when we incorporate them into our daily lives, we build strength, maintain flexibility and support long-term health. It's not about working out harder; it's about moving smarter in ways that feel natural and sustainable.

The Foundation of Movement – Strength, Flexibility and Mobility

Movement is life. Every action we take, whether it's standing, walking, lifting or even reaching for a glass of water, depends on a delicate balance between strength, flexibility and mobility. These three elements form the foundation of how well our bodies function, how efficiently we move and how resilient we remain as we age. While many people focus on just one aspect – strength training for muscles, or stretching for flexibility – the truth is, they work together as a system. Without strength, we lack stability. Without flexibility, we lose mobility. And without mobility, even daily movements can become difficult and painful.

In the next leg of our journey we will explore the science and practice of strength, flexibility and stretching, how they work, why they decline with age and most importantly, how you can maintain and improve them. By understanding these fundamental components, you'll be able to build a body that is strong, flexible and capable, one that moves effortlessly, stays resilient and supports you for a lifetime.

The Power of Strength: Why Your Muscles Matter More Than You Think

When people think of strength training, they often picture heavy weights or bulky muscles. But strength isn't just about appearance; it's about how well your body functions and supports you in everyday life. From getting up from a chair to carrying groceries or maintaining posture, your muscles play a vital role in every movement. And just like flexibility, strength naturally declines with age, unless you take steps to preserve it.

Though I've already mentioned it, it's worth repeating: After age 30, muscle mass starts to decrease by about 3–8 percent per decade. After 60, the decline can reach up to 15 percent per decade. This loss, known as sarcopenia, doesn't just make you weaker, it affects metabolism, bone health and even brain function. Without sufficient strength, daily tasks like walking, climbing stairs or keeping your balance become more difficult, raising the risk of falls and injuries.

Strength training, whether through bodyweight moves, resistance bands or lifting weights, helps maintain and even rebuild muscle mass. While cardio is great for heart and lung health, strength training targets your muscles directly, making them stronger and more resilient. And it's not just muscles that benefit; it also boosts bone density, lowering the risk of osteoporosis, and improves joint stability, to prevent injuries.

Many believe that walking or staying generally active is enough. While walking supports cardiovascular health, it doesn't challenge muscles the way strength training does. Our bodies are built for varied movement – pushing, pulling, squatting, lifting, carrying. These functional patterns reflect real-life actions and form the base of a capable, mobile body.

The great thing is, strength training doesn't require a gym or heavy equipment. Bodyweight exercises like squats, push-ups, lunges and planks are highly effective and can be done anywhere. If you prefer weights, light dumbbells or resistance bands work well too. The key is consistency – training at least two to three times per week with progressive overload, meaning gradually increasing resistance or intensity, ensures steady gains.

Interestingly, strength is deeply tied to longevity and overall health. Grip strength, for instance, is a strong indicator of lifespan. People with higher grip strength tend to live longer, have lower heart disease risk and retain better brain function with age. It's a reminder that maintaining strength isn't just about performance, but it's about health, vitality and independence too.

Another overlooked benefit of strength training is its effect on the brain. Resistance exercises boost growth factors that support memory, mood and cognitive health. Research even links strength training to a reduced risk of Alzheimer's and dementia, showing that a strong body supports a sharp mind.

So if you're looking for a simple, powerful way to boost your health, strength training is essential. It's not about becoming a bodybuilder or lifting huge weights; it's about staying strong enough to move with ease at every stage of life. Whether it's lifting, pushing or simply carrying your own weight, strength is the foundation of movement, health and longevity.

Here's the good news: strength loss isn't inevitable. It's one of the most preventable parts of ageing.

And the best part: It's never too late to start.

The Science and Practice of Flexibility and Stretching

Have you ever noticed how easily children can bend, squat and move in ways that seem impossible for many adults? That's because flexibility peaks in youth and naturally declines with age. It's something we rarely think about until we start feeling stiff, tight or restricted. But

Grip Strength: A Hidden Marker of Health

Grip strength is more than just a measure of how strong your hands are; it's a powerful indicator of overall health and longevity. It refers to the force your hand and forearm muscles can generate when gripping, holding or squeezing an object. Scientists have found that grip strength is closely linked to physical resilience, heart health and even brain function. A weak grip is often associated with an increased risk of falls, higher mortality rates and cognitive decline. In fact, studies suggest that grip strength may be a better predictor of lifespan than blood pressure! It is typically measured using a handheld device called a dynamometer, which records how much force you can apply. Fortunately, improving grip strength is simple and can be done through daily activities like carrying groceries, opening jars or squeezing a stress ball. More structured exercises, such as deadlifts, pull-ups and hanging from a bar can also enhance grip strength and overall muscle function. Training your grip isn't just about having a firm handshake – it's about maintaining strength, stability and independence as you age.

flexibility isn't just about touching your toes; it's essential for how we move, recover and manage pain and inflammation.

From early on, we each have different levels of flexibility. Some people feel naturally tight, while others are hyper-flexible and bend with ease. Neither extreme is ideal – too little flexibility can lead to stiffness and injury, while too much may cause joint instability. The key lies in maintaining a balanced range of motion that lets you move freely and comfortably.

The science behind flexibility is fascinating. It's not just about stretching muscles; it's about the coordination between your nervous system, muscles and connective tissues. When you stretch, your brain and nervous system actively decide how far you can go without risk. That's why flexibility isn't about forcing a stretch – it's about teaching your body to feel safe and supported in greater ranges of motion.

As we age, flexibility naturally decreases. Between ages 20 and 49, the decline is gradual. But after 50, it accelerates. Research shows we lose around 10 percent per decade. This is less about ageing itself and more about how our lifestyles change. We tend to move less, sit more and stick to repetitive motions that limit full-body mobility.

Not all stretching is the same. Static stretching – holding a position for a set time – is the most effective way to improve flexibility. Holding stretches for 30 to 60 seconds and doing them consistently, ideally five to seven times a week, brings the best results. Dynamic stretching – moving through full ranges of motion – is excellent for warming up before activity.

A balanced flexibility routine doesn't need extreme poses or hours of effort. It needs consistency: regular movement, mindful technique and a little patience. Whether you choose yoga, traditional stretching or a mix of both, flexibility work is one of the simplest, most effective ways to keep your body strong and youthful.

So next time you feel tight or stiff, remember, your body is made to move. And with a little daily effort, you can stay limber, agile and pain-free for years to come.

The good news: regular stretching and movement can slow or even reverse the decline in flexibility, keeping joints healthy and reducing injury risk.

After reading about strength, flexibility and mobility – knowing how vital movement is – are you now ready to plan your schedule? If yes, I can suggest a simple, effective formula to get started.

Practice FITT to Stay FIT!

FITT stands for **Frequency, Intensity, Time and Type** – A simple yet powerful formula to create an effective and sustainable exercise plan. Let's break it down step by step in a way that's practical and easy to apply in your daily life.

Frequency: How Often Do You Move?

1. How many times a week do you exercise?

Consistency is key! A single workout here and there won't do much for your health. To truly reap the benefits of exercise, you need to commit to a regular schedule. Whether you're practicing yoga or Pilates, hitting the gym or doing self-guided workouts, keep going! And if you haven't started yet – **don't wait, start today!**

2. How often do you move in a day?

Many people work out for an hour in the morning, then remain sedentary for the rest of the day. You may have heard the phrase 'Sitting is the new smoking'. It's not an exaggeration. Prolonged sitting has been linked to major health risks, including heart disease and metabolic disorders. If you sit for long hours, make sure to stand up every 90 to 120 minutes, stretch, twist, move and repeat.

What's the Ideal Frequency?

Aim for 5–6 days of structured exercise per week.

Avoid prolonged sitting; move every 90–120 minutes throughout the day.

Intensity: Find Your Balance

These days it's common to hear stories of people, including celebrities, collapsing in the gym. Why does this happen? Because they push themselves **too hard** without respecting their body's limits.

Exercise is not a battle against your body. Bend, don't break!

Avoid comparisons. Fitness is personal. Your body is unique and your workout should be tailored to your needs.

Find the right intensity based on your age, body type, fitness level and experience.

The key is progressive overload – challenge yourself gradually without overdoing it. Listen to your body and adjust your intensity as needed.

Time: Stretch Your Comfort Zone

How long should you exercise? Time plays a crucial role in defining the intensity and effectiveness of your workout.

If you can do 12 reps, try 15 next time.

If you can hold a yoga pose for 20 seconds, extend it to 25.

Progress gradually. Exercise should be mild to moderate, never excessive.

Aerobic Exercise (Cardio)

150–300 minutes of moderate-intensity or 75–150 minutes of vigorous-intensity exercise per week (WHO, 2020) is recommended.

Daily goal: At least 30 minutes of moderate activity (eg: brisk walking, cycling or swimming) 5 days a week.

Daily Step Count

Aim for at least 7,000–8,000 steps per day for better cardiovascular health and longevity (Paluch et al., JAMA, 2021).

Strength Training

At least two days per week, focussing on major muscle groups (AHA, 2018).

Daily goal: 10–15 minutes of strength training (eg: bodyweight workouts, resistance bands or weights).

Flexibility and Mobility

5–10 minutes of stretching daily to maintain flexibility and prevent injuries.

Your body improves when you gently push your limits over time, not through excessive strain but through consistent, progressive movement.

Type: What Should You Do?
The Answer? Do What You Love!

Exercise is a lifelong habit; to make it sustainable, it must be something you truly enjoy. A habit becomes part of your routine when it feels rewarding, easy to maintain and naturally appealing. Instead of forcing yourself into a workout you dislike, choose activities that align with your interests and lifestyle. Whether it's walking in nature, engaging in cardio sessions, practicing yoga for flexibility and mindfulness, hitting the gym for strength training, playing your favourite sport, swimming for a full-body workout or challenging yourself with high-intensity exercises, find what excites you. The key is variety; mixing different forms of exercise keeps it engaging and ensures a balanced approach to fitness. By choosing activities you love, you make movement a natural and enjoyable part of your daily life, setting the foundation for lifelong health and well-being.

Variety is Key

Repeating the same workout daily can lead to boredom and stagnation. Instead, mix it up. A varied routine keeps you engaged, prevents overuse injuries and challenges different muscles.

Incorporate the 7 Fundamental Human Movements

A well-rounded workout should include **basic movement patterns** to build functional strength and mobility. These movements are the foundation of all physical activities we do in daily life. Training them ensures a balanced, functional and strong body.

1. **Push (Pushing Movements):** Think of pushing a heavy door open or pressing something overhead. These types of movements

build upper body strength, especially in the chest, shoulders and arms. **Examples: Push-ups, Overhead Presses**

2. **Pull (Pulling Movements):** Imagine pulling a heavy bag toward you or opening a stubborn drawer. These strengthen the back, biceps and grip, improving posture and reducing back pain. **Examples: Rows, Pull-ups**
3. **Squat (Bending the Knees to Lower the Body):** Picture yourself sitting down in a chair and standing back up. That's a squat. There are excellent exercises to strengthen the legs, hips and core, making everyday movements like standing and lifting easier. **Examples: Bodyweight Squats, Goblet Squats**
4. **Hinge (Bending at the Hips):** Think of picking something up from the floor with a straight back – this is a hinge movement that strengthens the lower back, glutes and hamstrings, preventing injuries and improving posture. **Examples: Deadlifts, Hip Bridges**
5. **Lunge (Stepping Forward or Backward While Bending the Knees):** Imagine taking a big step forward or kneeling down to tie your shoes. Benefits of these are to improve balance, coordination and leg strength, making walking and climbing stairs easier. **Examples: Forward Lunges, Split Squats**
6. **Twist (Rotational Movements):** Picture twisting your body to grab something from the back seat of a car. It works the core muscles, especially the obliques, and improves flexibility in the spine. **Examples: Russian Twists, Spinal Rotations**
7. **Gait (Locomotion – Moving Your Body from One Place to Another):** This includes all forms of movement like walking, running and even crawling (yes, crawling is a great exercise!). This are essential for overall mobility, endurance and heart health. **Examples: Walking, Running, Crawling**

These seven movements mimic natural human motions and are essential for strength, balance and injury prevention. Training using them regularly ensures your body moves efficiently in everyday life, reducing strain and keeping you active and pain-free. A balanced programme that incorporates all these movements will improve strength, flexibility and overall mobility.

Do what you love. Keep your workouts varied. Make movement a lifelong habit!

The Soleus Muscle: Your Hidden Metabolic Powerhouse

Walking & the Soleus: The Forgotten Connection

Walking is often praised as one of the best forms of exercise, but have you ever thought about the muscles that make it possible? The soleus, a deep calf muscle, plays a major role. It helps maintain posture, supports endurance and aids circulation. Each step you take activates the soleus, propelling you forward and pumping blood back to the heart.

Unlike the more prominent gastrocnemius, which helps in jumping and sprinting, the soleus is your slow-twitch endurance muscle, working steadily when you walk or stand. But there's more: recent research shows that it also plays a key role in regulating blood sugar, making it critical for metabolic health.

Why the Soleus Muscle is Unique

The soleus stands out in the muscular system. It supports movement, metabolism and circulation, yet is often overlooked. One of its standout traits is endurance. Made mostly of slow-twitch fibres, the soleus works continuously without tiring, whether you're standing, walking or just holding posture.

Its energy-burning ability is equally impressive. Unlike many muscles that rely on stored glycogen, the soleus prefers to pull glucose directly from the blood. This makes it especially effective for managing blood sugar – an advantage for people with insulin resistance or diabetes.

It's also vital for circulation. Often called a 'secondary heart', the soleus helps push blood from the lower legs back up to the heart, reducing the risk of pooling, varicose veins and deep vein thrombosis.

What's even more fascinating is that the soleus can help control blood sugar, without needing insulin. This means that activating it can naturally regulate glucose, without the body relying on medication.

Soleus and Glucose Uptake: A Metabolic Breakthrough

Recent research by Mark Hamilton et al (2022) uncovered a powerful fact: The soleus can burn glucose directly from the bloodstream without insulin. This could be a game-changer for managing blood sugar and improving metabolic health.

Unlike other muscles that use stored glycogen, the soleus taps into circulating glucose and fat. Activating it helps lower blood sugar levels, even in people with insulin resistance.

Here's what the research found:

- **Soleus activation boosts glucose uptake by 52 percent,** even at low intensity. You don't need high-intensity workouts; simple movements activate it effectively.
- **It keeps working for hours without fatigue.** Unlike most muscles, the soleus continues burning glucose long after you've stopped moving.
- **It reduces insulin resistance.** Because it works independently of insulin, it offers a natural way to regulate blood sugar without taxing the pancreas.
- **It supports fat metabolism.** By efficiently burning fat, it helps prevent fat buildup and supports better energy balance.

These findings highlight how powerful – and often ignored – the soleus truly is. Activities like walking, soleus push-ups or seated heel raises can activate it and unlock its benefits. For better blood sugar control, fat metabolism and overall health, focussing on the soleus may be one of the simplest and most effective strategies.

Despite all this, the soleus is rarely targeted in standard fitness routines. By incorporating movements like walking, calf raises and soleus push-ups, you can activate this metabolic powerhouse and support your circulation, energy and well-being.

How to Strengthen the Soleus Muscle

Soleus Push-Ups (SPUs) – The Secret to Glucose Control

A simple, seated exercise that stimulates the soleus for long-lasting metabolic benefits: Sit with feet flat on the ground and knees at 90 degrees.

Keep your toes on the floor and lift your heels slowly.

Lower your heels back down in a controlled motion.

Repeat for 30-60 minutes intermittently throughout the day.

Unlike traditional exercises, SPUs are effective even when sitting, making them easy to incorporate into daily life.

Seated Soleus Raises (Seated Calf Raises) – Best for Strength

Sit on a chair with feet flat on the ground.

Place a weight (or your hands) on your knees.

Lift your heels off the ground, keeping knees bent.

Lower slowly and repeat.

Isolates the soleus and removes the gastrocnemius from the movement.

Walking and Stair Climbing – Everyday Activation

Walking naturally activates the soleus, but adding inclines or stairs increases its engagement.

Aim for 7,000–8,000 steps per day for optimal metabolic benefits.

Calf Size as an Indicator of Health

The size and strength of your calf muscles can indicate overall metabolic and cardiovascular health. Research suggests that larger, stronger calves are linked to better circulation, improved glucose metabolism and reduced risk of vascular diseases.

How to Measure Your Calf Health

Use your thumb and index finger from both hands to encircle your calf: If your index fingers and thumbs touch in front, your calf size is proportionate.

If your fingers do not touch, your calf size is strong and well-developed.

If your fingers overlap significantly, it may indicate weaker calf muscles.

Now compare this with your neck and abdominal circumference. Measure your neck in the same way; it should be less than your calf circumference. Measure your abdomen by placing your thumbs at your spine and index fingers at your sides, then moving them toward your navel. Your waist should be equal to or less than twice the size of your calf circumference.

This simple assessment can help you determine if your body proportions are balanced for optimal metabolic and postural health.

The soleus muscle is not just a walking muscle – it is a metabolic powerhouse that regulates blood sugar, improves circulation and supports endurance. Whether through Soleus Push-Ups, seated calf raises or simply walking, engaging this muscle can provide long-term health benefits.

Yoga *Asanas* – The Healing Power of Movement

Yoga *asanas*, those graceful postures seen in yoga classes, are far more than exercises. They're powerful tools for physical and mental healing. When we enter a yoga posture, we're not just stretching muscles, we're engaging the deep intelligence of the nervous system. Have you noticed your body sometimes resists a stretch? That's your nervous system protecting you. But with conscious breathing and relaxation, the body learns to release, allowing greater mobility over time. This is why regular yoga practitioners often feel more flexible, experience less pain and handle stress more effectively.

What Makes an *Asana* Special?

The word *asana* means 'posture', but it's not just any posture; it's one held with awareness and control. Unlike random daily movements, *asanas* are intentional. Each involves entering the pose, holding it mindfully and exiting with control. The magic lies in the holding. When we stay in a pose with awareness, something powerful happens.

Muscles stretch, while opposing muscles contract, creating gentle tension that stimulates nerves and blood vessels. This mild stress sends signals to the brain, awakening the body's healing systems. Think of it as a soft alarm that guides attention to areas needing care. That's why yoga feels therapeutic; it brings balance and encourages recovery.

Yoga, when practiced with awareness, becomes deeply healing. It's not about forcing flexibility or mastering difficult poses. Therapeutic yoga restores balance and works with the body's natural healing ability. Moving gently and breathing deeply improves circulation, eases tension and enhances nerve function. This is especially helpful for chronic pain, stiffness or injury recovery.

The Sixth Sense: Proprioception

One of yoga's most intriguing effects is how it sharpens *proprioception* – our sense of body position and movement. Even with your eyes closed, you know where your limbs are. That's proprioception at work.

Proprioceptors are tiny sensors in muscles, tendons and joints that constantly send feedback to the brain about body position. This internal GPS helps us move smoothly, stay balanced and avoid injury. Walking in the dark without stumbling? That's thanks to proprioceptors.

Yoga fine-tunes this sense. In poses like Tree or Warrior, proprioceptors are fully engaged, helping you stay balanced and stable. That's why yoga improves coordination, reaction time and overall balance. For athletes, dancers and those healing from injuries, building proprioception through yoga is a true asset.

Practicing yoga challenges your sense of movement in a safe, controlled way. Some poses demand stillness, others involve flow, but all activate proprioceptors and train the nervous system to respond better.

So don't hesitate to step onto your mat. Remember: You're not just moving. You're tuning in, communicating with your body and awakening your inner healing intelligence.

References

1. Bouchard, C., Blair, S. N., & Haskell, W. L. (2012). *Physical Activity and Health*. Human Kinetics.
2. Frontera, W. R., Hughes, V. A., Lutz, K. J., & Evans, W. J. (1991). A cross-sectional study of muscle strength and mass in 45- to 78-yr-old men and women. *Journal of Applied Physiology, 71*(2), 644–650. https://doi.org/10.1152/jappl.1991.71.2.644
3. Fleg, J. L., & Lakatta, E. G. (1988). Role of muscle loss in the age-associated reduction in VO2 max. *Journal of Applied Physiology, 65*(3), 1147–1151. https://doi.org/10.1152/jappl.1988.65.3.1147
4. Lee, I. M., Shiroma, E. J., Lobelo, F., Puska, P., Blair, S. N., & Katzmarzyk, P. T. (2012). Effect of physical inactivity on major non-communicable diseases worldwide: An analysis of burden of disease and life expectancy. *The Lancet, 380*(9838), 219–229. https://doi.org/10.1016/S0140-6736(12)61031-9
5. Bohannon, R. W. (2019). Grip strength: An indispensable biomarker for older adults. *Clinical Interventions in Aging, 14*, 1681–1691. https://doi.org/10.2147/CIA.S194543

6. Larson, E. B., Wang, L., Bowen, J. D., McCormick, W. C., Teri, L., Crane, P., & Kukull, W. (2006). Exercise is associated with reduced risk for incident dementia among persons 65 years of age and older. *Annals of Internal Medicine, 144*(2), 73–81. https://doi.org/10.7326/0003-4819-144-2-200601170-00004
7. Warburton, D. E. R., Nicol, C. W., & Bredin, S. S. D. (2006). Health benefits of physical activity: The evidence. *Canadian Medical Association Journal, 174*(6), 801–809. https://doi.org/10.1503/cmaj.051351
8. Paluch, A. E., Bajpai, S., Bassett, D. R., Carnethon, M. R., Ekelund, U., Evenson, K. R., ... & Kraus, W. E. (2022). Daily steps and all-cause mortality: A meta-analysis. *JAMA Network Open, 5*(9), e2238016. https://doi.org/10.1001/jamanetworkopen.2022.38016
9. World Health Organization. (2020). *WHO guidelines on physical activity and sedentary behavior.*
10. Paluch, A. E., et al. (2021). *Daily steps and all-cause mortality: a meta-analysis.* JAMA.
11. American Heart Association. (2018). *Recommendations for physical activity in adults.*

CHAPTER 6
The Mystery

Mind: The Whisper Left Unheard!

Mind: The Mystery

The chicken-or-egg debate may one day be solved, but the mind's nature and location might always remain elusive. Instead of getting stuck on what or where the mind is, it's more helpful to recognise its vital role in health, disease and well-being. The mind can be both a friend and a foe. What matters is how we use it to our benefit.

Have you ever wondered why the mind creates discomfort or even illness? Is it even real? Let's rewind to childhood. Many of us, or our friends, have experienced an upset stomach just before an exam. It often came out of nowhere, right before a test. Why? Because the body responds to stress. When we anticipate something stressful – like an exam we're not prepared for – our body seeks escape. The easiest way? A physical symptom. A stomach ache offers both distraction and, possibly, a way out of the situation, like skipping the exam. In that moment, physical discomfort seems more manageable than anxiety.

But it doesn't stop there. Because the stomach ache 'worked', the body starts adopting this as a coping mechanism. Over time, this becomes a pattern. Stress triggers physical symptoms like headaches, cramps, even blackouts. Eventually, your brain perceives even mild pressure – an interview, a presentation or simply imagining a challenge – as a real threat. The body, having learned that symptoms can offer relief, keeps using that strategy.

The problem is that what starts as a simple stomach ache can escalate into long-term issues. Constant stress responses may disrupt digestion, leading to bloating, acidity, IBS or even autoimmune conditions. Chronic headaches, muscle tension, high blood pressure and a weakened immune system can ensue. The cycle becomes self-reinforcing – stress causes symptoms, and the symptoms create more stress.

This story highlights the deep mind-body connection. What we think and feel often becomes physical. Our thoughts shape reality, not just metaphorically, but biologically. When we think better, we feel better. And when we feel better, we act better. The way we perceive events shapes how the body responds. Two people can face the same situation but react entirely differently, depending on their mindset.

A simple example is a child scared of their shadow. They run, screaming, convinced something dark is chasing them. We laugh because we know it's harmless. But the child's fear is real. Perhaps someone told them darkness is scary, or their mind filled the unknown with fear. Adults do the same – we fear the unknown more than actual events. Like the child, we react to uncertainty with stress.

When we're stressed, the body activates its fight-or-flight mode. This goes back to our hunter-gatherer ancestors. Imagine walking in a forest and spotting a lion. The body instantly prepares, pumping blood to muscles, increasing heart rate, shutting down digestion. If you survive, the body resets, relaxes and heals. And if you encounter another danger later, the cycle repeats. No harm done as long as there's recovery in between.

But in today's world, we don't meet lions; we face deadlines, conflicts, financial worries. The stress isn't short-lived. It lingers. And this keeps our fight-or-flight system constantly activated. The result? Chronic high blood pressure, shallow breathing, fatigue, digestion problems, anxiety, panic and long-term illness. Our bodies were made for short bursts of stress, not endless tension.

Another problem is decision-making. When facing a lion, we don't think, we act. But modern problems need thought and reasoning. Yet, under stress, the brain pushes us toward instinctive, often irrational choices. That's why we make poor decisions when overwhelmed, trapped in a stress loop.

So what's the way out? The answer lies in activating the body's rest-and-heal mode, run by the parasympathetic nervous system. We must guide our bodies back to calm, the way our ancestors did after surviving danger.

Understanding the root of stress and how it affects both mind and body is the first step toward healing. When we shift from survival mode to restoration, we create space for clarity, vitality and health. This is exactly what we do in Naturopathy & Yoga healing centres – we support the body's natural ability to rest, recover and restore.

The Rest and Heal Mechanism

Think of the sympathetic nervous system as the accelerator of a car, and the parasympathetic system as the brakes. We need both for the car to function properly, but we can only use one at a time. If we keep pressing the accelerator without ever applying the brakes, the car will crash. This is exactly what happens when stress dominates our lives. Our system is constantly in overdrive, unable to slow down and heal.

The parasympathetic nervous system (PNS) is responsible for activating the body's natural rest-and-heal mode. It is also referred to as the 'rest and digest' system and counterbalances the fight-or-flight response by slowing heart rate, reducing blood pressure, enhancing digestion and promoting deep relaxation. When the PNS is engaged, the body enters a state of repair, allowing healing processes to function optimally.

The PNS controls vital functions such as the vocal cords, optimal heart function, lung capacity, liver and digestive processes, bladder control and reproductive system health. This is why, under acute or extreme stress or fear, people may temporarily lose their voice, experience heart palpitations or even lose bladder control. Chronic stress and prolonged activation of the sympathetic nervous system suppress the parasympathetic response, leading to conditions like digestive disorders, weakened immunity and chronic fatigue. Restoring balance by activating the PNS is crucial for long-term health. A well-functioning parasympathetic nervous system ensures that the body has adequate time to repair and regenerate. Without it, healing becomes compromised, increasing the risk of chronic diseases. By understanding and nurturing this vital system, we can reclaim our natural ability to heal and thrive.

Naturopathy & Yoga healing work by activating the parasympathetic system, allowing the body to switch into its natural repair mode. When this happens, healing is no longer forced; it happens naturally, as was always designed.

Naturopathic Approaches to Activating the Parasympathetic Nervous System (PNS)

In a Naturopathy hospital we use various techniques that work on the body to indirectly influence the brain and activate the parasympathetic nervous system. Yogic breathing practices such as deep breathing, OM chanting and singing (*keerthans* and *bhajans*) play a vital role. Yogic Kriyas like Laghu Shankha Prakshalana and Dhauti further support this process. Aromatherapy is another effective tool, known for its calming effects on the nervous system.

One of the most well-known naturopathic treatments is hydrotherapy, where cold or alternating hot and cold applications help trigger the body's relaxation response. Many of these techniques can be easily incorporated into daily life once properly learned under the guidance of a Naturopathy doctor. However, some treatments, like specific Yogic Kriyas and advanced hydrotherapy techniques, require professional supervision and are best practiced in a controlled setting at a Naturopathy hospital.

The Power of Deep Breathing

Deep breathing is one of the simplest and most effective ways to activate the body's relaxation response. From childhood, we instinctively tell someone who is angry, agitated, or nervous to "chill" and "take a deep breath". But have you ever wondered why this works? The answer lies in a simple psychological and physiological principle: 'fake it till you make it'.When we are in a naturally relaxed state, our breathing slows down and becomes deeper. But what if we consciously breathe in this way when we are stressed? The body does not distinguish whether we are truly relaxed or just mimicking the breathing pattern. It simply assumes relaxation is happening and, in response, activates the parasympathetic nervous system. This means that even during stressful situations, maintaining a deep, steady breathing rhythm can shift the body out of a stress response and into a state of calm.

However, there's a practical question – can we consciously practice deep breathing when we are in the middle of extreme stress, such as road rage? The answer is likely no. But that does not make deep breathing any less useful. Consider this: We do not wait to learn swimming until we accidentally fall into water, right? We equip ourselves beforehand, practicing in a controlled environment so that if the situation arises, we know how to handle it. The same principle applies to deep breathing. By practicing it regularly, we train our bodies to maintain slow, steady breathing even in stressful conditions, making it an automatic response rather than a forced effort.

Deep breathing is effective not just because it mimics a relaxed state, but also because it directly engages the diaphragm, a dome-shaped muscle below the lungs. The diaphragm is closely connected to the parasympathetic nervous system. When we take slow, deep breaths that engage the diaphragm we stimulate the vagus nerve, which plays a crucial role in activating the body's relaxation response.

A simple way to practice deep breathing is to sit or lie down comfortably, place one hand on the belly, and breathe in deeply through the nose. The goal is to allow the abdomen to expand while keeping the chest as still as possible. A key trick to enhance relaxation is making the exhalation longer than the inhalation, as this signals the nervous system to relax even further.

THE DIAPHRAGM FUNCTIONS IN BREATHING

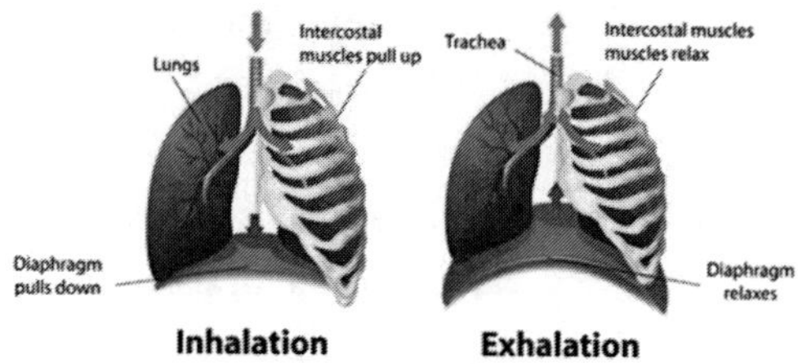

OM Chanting and Singing: Activating the Vagus Nerve

OM chanting and singing work effectively in multiple ways. One reason is that our sound box – the larynx – is supplied by a branch of the vagus nerve, which plays a key role in the parasympathetic nervous system. When we exert mild stress on the larynx through vocalisation, it activates the parasympathetic branch to restore balance.

Vibrational sounds, like humming, chanting 'OM', or singing have a calming effect on the body because they naturally stimulate the vagus nerve – a key nerve that helps regulate relaxation, digestion and overall well-being. The vagus nerve runs from the brain down to the heart, lungs and digestive system, and its job is to shift the body into 'rest and heal' mode by lowering stress, slowing heart rate and improving digestion.

When you hum, chant or sing, the vibrations from your voice travel through your throat, chest and head. These vibrations gently massage and activate the vagus nerve, sending signals to the brain that everything is safe and relaxed. As a result the body releases fewer stress hormones, muscles loosen up and a sense of calm takes over.

Scientific studies show that chanting or singing regularly can help lower blood pressure, reduce anxiety and even improve mood by increasing feel-good chemicals like serotonin and oxytocin. That's why people often feel peaceful after singing in a choir, chanting *mantras* or even just humming a tune they love.

How Exercise Supports the 'Rest and Heal' Mode

Exercises and movements not only work in the body but also in the mind. If you're someone who enjoys exercise, you've probably felt that sense of happiness or calm after a workout. Some call it a 'runner's high', but it's not just for joggers – any form of movement can bring about that feel-good sensation. This happens because exercise activates not only our muscles, but also our nervous system and hormones, shifting us toward relaxation and recovery.

When we engage in physical activity, especially mindful movement like yoga, stretching or even a simple walk, we are helping balance our autonomic nervous system – the system that controls involuntary functions like heart rate, digestion and breathing. Gentle movement, combined with deep, controlled breathing, signals the body that it is safe, reducing stress and promoting a shift from the fight-or-flight response to a calmer state.

Certain restorative yoga poses, such as child's pose or supported backbends, help activate the parasympathetic nervous system by reducing tension in key areas like the spine, diaphragm and abdomen. Walking, especially in nature, has been shown to lower cortisol (the stress hormone) and improve mental clarity. The rhythmic movement of walking or yoga, paired with breath awareness, gently guides the nervous system toward relaxation.

The Healing Power of Aromatherapy

Have you ever smelled something and instantly been reminded of a memory? Maybe the scent of fresh cookies takes you back to childhood, or a certain perfume brings someone special to mind.

That's because our sense of smell is deeply connected to our emotions and memories – it's incredibly powerful. This is the essence of aromatherapy: using scents to influence our body and mind in meaningful ways.

Smelling something isn't just about enjoying pleasant fragrances. When we inhale a scent, tiny molecules travel through our nose to special receptors that send signals directly to the brain, specifically the limbic system. This part of the brain governs emotions, memory and behaviour. That's why some smells make us feel calm, energised or nostalgic.

Essential oils are natural plant extracts that have been used for centuries to promote health and well-being. These oils impact the nervous system, which regulates heart rate, digestion and stress. Inhaling essential oils prompts the brain to release feel-good chemicals. For instance, lavender boosts serotonin and GABA, helping reduce stress and aid sleep. Citrus oils like orange and lemon enhance dopamine and serotonin levels, improving mood, focus and energy.

The beauty of aromatherapy is its simplicity. Using a diffuser is one of the easiest ways to enjoy the benefits, spreading the scent into the air for natural inhalation. Oils can also be applied topically, when diluted with a carrier oil like coconut or almond oil and massaged onto pulse points such as wrists, temples or neck. Direct inhalation – taking a deep breath from a bottle or using a drop on a tissue – offers quick relief from stress or headaches. Adding essential oils to a warm bath or a damp cloth can deepen relaxation and ease muscle tension.

Different essential oils serve different therapeutic purposes. Lavender is famous for calming the mind and aiding sleep. Chamomile soothes stress and supports digestion. Peppermint energises and eases headaches. Sandalwood is grounding and improves mental clarity. Eucalyptus helps clear sinuses and strengthen immunity. Lemon uplifts mood and boosts concentration.

Research backs aromatherapy's benefits. Studies show that inhaling essential oils can lower cortisol (stress hormone), reduce blood pressure and heart rate, promote melatonin production for better sleep, support immunity and help ease anxiety and depression. Aromatherapy is a natural, effective way to support well-being. Whether you want to relax, lift your mood or sharpen focus, there's an essential oil that can help. So the next time you need a reset or a moment of calm, take a deep breath and let nature work its magic.

Enemas: The Unsung Heroes of Naturopathy

Enemas are often misunderstood and overlooked in modern healing methods, yet they have been an essential part of traditional and naturopathic medicine for centuries. Many people feel awkward about enemas, and I was no exception. As a Naturopathy & Yoga medical student, in my college days I made a firm decision: When I started my clinical practice, I would never recommend enemas because they seemed uncomfortable and embarrassing. However, I soon realised how foolish that thought was.

Enemas are an incredibly effective way to promote relaxation by improving gut health. Contrary to popular belief, the purpose of an enema is not merely to insert 500 ml of water into the rectum and flush out waste. The benefits go far beyond simple cleansing. The gut and brain are intricately connected through the vagus nerve, and cleansing the colon helps reduce inflammation and supports parasympathetic activation. This process promotes relaxation, detoxification and overall well-being.

When the colon is cleansed, the reduction of accumulated toxins and irritation leads to a decrease in gut inflammation, which in turn helps signal the brain to shift from a stress state to a relaxed state. The gentle stimulation of the rectal nerves during an enema can also directly activate the vagus nerve, further enhancing PNS activity. This results in improved digestion, a calmer nervous system and better overall well-being.

While enemas can be self-administered with proper training, it is always best to undergo the process under the guidance of a trained

Naturopathy expert. Various healing traditions incorporate enemas in different ways, both medicated and non-medicated. In Naturopathy, we generally prefer non-medicated enemas, adjusting the temperature based on the individual's condition and needs. However, at times, specific herbal enemas, such as those using neem, tender coconut water or coffee, are recommended for their therapeutic properties.

The practice of enemas, when done correctly, can aid in detoxification, relieve constipation, support liver function and help restore balance to the digestive system. By activating the parasympathetic nervous system, enemas contribute to deep relaxation, improved gut function and overall nervous system harmony. Despite the initial hesitation some may feel, enemas remain one of the most powerful tools in natural healing, offering benefits that extend far beyond gut health.

Yogic Kriyas: Cleansing Procedures in Yoga

Yoga is a vast ocean, offering something for everyone. Among its many aspects, Yogic Kriyas hold a special place in promoting both physical and mental well-being. These cleansing techniques not only purify the body, but influence the mind, fostering harmony and balance. Laghu Shankha Prakshalana and Dhauti are especially powerful for supporting body-mind healing, particularly through their impact on the gastrointestinal tract and the parasympathetic nervous system (PNS).

It's truly fascinating how these ancient practices align so well with modern scientific understanding. For those unfamiliar, they may initially seem intimidating, but that changes with experience. As mentioned in earlier chapters, naturopathic healing is a process of empowerment, and learning these techniques is part of that journey. They help us connect directly with internal systems that are typically beyond conscious control. Interestingly, most of these transformative practices require only water, salt and proper technique – skills that are easy to learn. Let's explore two *kriyas* that reveal the power of this cleansing system.

Laghu Shankha Prakshalana: This traditional yogic technique involves drinking warm saline water followed by specific yoga postures to cleanse the digestive tract. By eliminating accumulated waste and toxins, it enhances gut health and strengthens the gut-brain connection, leading to deeper relaxation. A clean digestive system supports optimal body function, promoting mental clarity, emotional stability and calm.

While effective, this *kriya* should not be overdone, ideally practiced just once every six months. In Naturopathy hospitals, it's commonly used as part of a structured treatment plan.

Dhauti: Dhauti includes various techniques for clearing toxins from the digestive tract and restoring internal balance. One well-known version, Vamana Dhauti, involves drinking warm saline water and inducing vomiting to eliminate excess mucus and impurities from the stomach.

Some Dhauti practices are simple enough to learn once under guidance and then continue independently. Others require ongoing supervision until proficiency is gained to prevent complications.

Both Laghu Shankha Prakshalana and Dhauti profoundly affect the parasympathetic nervous system by improving vagal tone. By cleansing the gut and supporting digestion, they enhance the body's ability to shift from stress (sympathetic dominance) to relaxation (parasympathetic activation). This shift promotes detoxification, reduces anxiety, supports emotional balance and nurtures inner calm and healing.

Naturopathic therapies like hydrotherapy and massage further support the body's innate 'rest and heal' response. These treatments boost circulation, ease stress and encourage deep relaxation, all of which help the body restore and heal.

Hydrotherapy uses water at varying temperatures to stimulate circulation, ease muscle tension and enhance detoxification. Cold water invigorates the nervous system and builds resilience, while warm water relaxes the body and supports restful healing.

Massage therapy helps release muscle tension, improve lymphatic flow and lower stress hormones. It enhances oxygen and nutrient delivery to tissues, supporting cellular repair and overall vitality.

Meditation: Training the Mind to Heal the Body

For those unfamiliar, meditation is often mistaken for passive stillness. But in truth, it's one of the most powerful tools to rewire the brain. Meditation isn't just about staying calm in peaceful settings; it's about staying centred even in the midst of stress.

With regular practice, meditation helps shift us from being reaction-oriented to being action-oriented. What does that mean? Instead of reacting impulsively, you learn to pause and choose a response that truly serves you.

Take for example a situation where someone hits the back of your car. If you're reaction-oriented, you might step out angrily, yell and let your stress skyrocket. The conflict may escalate, possibly landing you in legal trouble, all triggered by someone else's error.

Now picture the same event, but with an action-oriented mindset. You stay calm, move the car to the side, check for damage, speak reasonably and possibly walk away with a simple handshake. The situation is the same, but your response transforms it into something manageable and calm, instead of chaotic.

If you're wondering how to begin meditating, it's like asking what shirt size fits best; the answer is personal. But a good starting point is simply being aware of your breath and thoughts.

Meditation isn't a fixed destination; it's a journey. While many paths exist – *tantras, chakras, mantras* – the most constant guide is the ***swara*: your breath**. It's been with you since birth.

Think of meditation as floating down a river. The smoother the current, the easier the journey. As the saying goes, 'Slow is smooth, and smooth is fast'. When breath slows, it steadies the mind. And in that stillness, depth arises – deep, relaxed, rhythmic breathing that flows effortlessly like gentle waves.

With each breath, awareness deepens. There's no force, no resistance, just quiet rhythm and mindful presence. This is breathwork in essence: slow, deep, complete, relaxed and rhythmic, carried by awareness.

To begin, you don't need a special space. Sit comfortably. Pay attention to your breath, its depth and rhythm. When your mind drifts, gently bring it back. This redirection is part of the practice. No judgement, just return to your breath again and again.

This simple practice is a powerful foundation. From here, you can explore other techniques, including guided meditations, to move from a 'mind full' state to a 'mindful' one. Even a few minutes daily can yield profound, lasting effects, making meditation a vital support in the body's natural healing journey.

Laughter: The Melody of Healing and Joy

'Where laughter echoes, heart find their home'

Someone's whatsapp status

Laughter is often called nature's best medicine, and for good reason. There's a saying that 'cheap and best' is a myth, but laughter proves otherwise. Think about the last time you laughed your lungs out. Remember how good you felt afterwards? That sense of joy and ease isn't just in your mind; it reflects a real biochemical shift in the body. Laughter releases endorphins – your body's natural painkillers – and lowers cortisol levels, which helps ease stress. It also improves circulation and boosts heart health. More importantly, it activates the parasympathetic nervous system, helping the body shift from stress into relaxation and healing.

From a naturopathic perspective, laughter is one of the simplest and most powerful tools to support health and well-being. It aligns beautifully with the body's innate healing intelligence by promoting balance and harmony. When you laugh, your immune system gets a natural boost, producing more immune cells and antibodies to help guard against illness. It also enhances oxygenation and circulation, aiding detoxification. Deep belly laughter works like an internal massage, relieving muscle tension, expanding lung capacity and encouraging calm. Much like hydrotherapy, deep breathing or sleep, laughter is a natural stress reliever.

Physiologically, laughter helps regulate stress hormones. In today's fast-paced world, chronic stress is linked to many health problems, from digestive issues to heart disease. Laughter lowers cortisol and adrenaline, reducing the toll of ongoing stress. At the same time, it stimulates the brain, enhancing clarity and cognitive function. It also boosts dopamine and serotonin, lifting mood and restoring emotional balance. As a result, laughter improves sleep quality and digestion. A calm mind naturally supports better digestion, easing discomfort and bloating.

Holistic healing recognises the deep connection between mind, body and spirit, and laughter is a wonderfully accessible way to nurture that connection. It requires no tools, no preparation, just a spark of joy and playfulness. Whether it's sharing a light moment with a friend, watching a funny video or seeing humour in everyday life, laughter is a daily prescription for better health.

By reading this, you might wonder, "What should I laugh about?" The best thing to laugh at is your own mistakes! We all do plenty of silly things worth laughing at, like taking things more seriously than needed, punishing ourselves for others' faults, letting emotions hijack us or allowing others to control our moods. Before bed, take a moment to recall these small things, make light of them and have a good laugh. Not only will this help you unwind, it will also remind you to let go of unnecessary burdens. Laughter is a gift – embrace it and let it heal you in the most natural way.

The Power of Connection: Why Social Bonds Heal

We're not meant to go through life alone. As humans, we are wired for connection, with other people, family, animals and nature. It's in our biology. Whether we like it or not, research proves that strong social bonds aren't just nice to have, they're essential for our health.

But let's be real: relationships aren't always smooth. Not every connection is comforting or uplifting, and inviting others into our lives often comes with a bit of chaos. Maybe it's the friend who tests your patience, the relative who always has an opinion or the emotional complexity of love and community. But that's the nature of connection. It means stepping out of our comfort zones, sharing experiences and embracing the messiness of human interaction. That's how we build belonging.

A few years ago, an elderly Italian man came to our centre. He had lost his wife and in his words, life had been "fading away". His children were busy, and he'd withdrawn into loneliness. After some gentle encouragement, he started attending the daily gatherings. It wasn't an instant transformation, but slowly, something changed. He laughed more. His posture straightened. He began telling stories again. When I asked what had shifted, he simply said, "I remembered I was alive." Science confirms this – loneliness is as harmful to health as smoking 15 cigarettes a day. The antidote? Connection.

Think of yourself as a puzzle piece, unique on your own, but part of a bigger picture. Wholeness comes when we form meaningful bonds, when we accept others and allow them to accept us. This isn't just poetic; it's biological.

When we deeply connect with others, our brains release oxytocin – the 'love' or 'bonding' hormone. It's the same chemical released when a mother holds her baby or when people share moments of trust. Oxytocin doesn't just feel good, it lowers cortisol, the stress hormone that fuels inflammation, anxiety and disease. Research shows people with strong social ties recover faster from illness, heal quicker and live longer. One famous Harvard study that followed people for over 80 years found that close relationships – not wealth, fame or even genetics – were the clearest predictors of a long, healthy, happy life.

On the flip side, loneliness is toxic. It's not just an emotion, it's a biological stressor. Disconnection triggers a survival response in the nervous system, keeping the body in low-grade stress. This elevates blood pressure, weakens immunity and raises the risk of heart disease, stroke and Alzheimer's. One study from Brigham Young University found that loneliness increases the risk of early death by 26 percent.

But connection is about more than avoiding illness; it's about thriving. Have you noticed how being around positive, supportive people makes you feel lighter? There's a reason. Connection regulates emotions, boosts immunity and even reduces pain. Studies show chronic pain patients with strong social support report less pain and recover faster than those who feel isolated.

Still, connection isn't about numbers; it's about depth. You can be surrounded by people and still feel alone if the relationships lack meaning. Healing happens when we're open, when we share, when we're vulnerable. It happens when we stop pretending we've got it all together and let others in, imperfections and all.

I once worked with a woman named Anuradha from Bangalore, India. She had been battling depression for years. While our centre helped her improve, she hadn't fully emerged from it by the time she left. As part of her follow-up, she began volunteering at a community group connected to a temple. At first, it was just a few hours weekly, but gradually she formed real bonds, not just with volunteers, but with the wider community. She described it as "waking up" after years of numbness. Her symptoms didn't ease because of a miracle cure, but because she rediscovered purpose and connection.

Here's the beautiful part: Connection doesn't have to be complicated. It could be calling a friend, joining a group or making space for meaningful conversations. Even small moments – a smile, a shared laugh, a kind word – can lift mood and create ripples of healing.

In a world that often glorifies independence, it's easy to forget how deeply we need each other. But healing isn't a solo journey. It happens between us, in the warmth of shared moments and the quiet assurance that we're not alone. Connection isn't just good for the heart; it's essential for healing.

Mind Healing Modalities

While self-practices are essential in the journey of mind-body healing, there are times when external guidance becomes necessary, especially to help with healing of the mind. At Naturopathy healing centres, a variety of techniques are employed depending on the physician's expertise and approach. Among these, counselling, Yogic philosophy, Neuro-Linguistic Programming (NLP) and Inner Child Healing are powerful tools for transforming the mind and fostering healing. So it is important to get a deep understanding of the various aspects of our 'Mind'.

In psychology, the term 'mind' is broad and general. However, Yoga offers a more refined understanding through the concept of *Antahkarana,* the 'Inner Instrument', composed of four key faculties. Recognising and working with these aspects enables a naturopathic physician to guide patients more effectively through the healing process.

1. **Manas (Thinking Mind)** – mind is like a bodyguard. Its job is to keep you safe, secure and alive. It constantly scans for threats,

creates thoughts to protect you and reacts based on past experiences. That's great for survival, but if you rely on it for growth and fulfilment, it's like asking your security guard to run your company. The mind isn't designed for big-picture thinking; it's wired for protection, which often means keeping you in your comfort zone, even when it's not serving you.

2. **Buddhi (Intellect)** – *Buddhi* is the decision-maker. Unlike the mind, which reacts, the intellect analyses, contemplates and helps you make conscious choices. When the intellect is in charge, it can use the mind's thoughts as tools rather than letting them run the show. This balance is key – let the mind handle security, but let the intellect lead the way toward wisdom, creativity and real growth.
3. **Ahamkara (Ego)** – *Ahamkara* gives us a sense of 'I' or 'me'. It shapes identity and personal boundaries, helping us function in society. But when it dominates, it fosters attachment, pride and rigidity. The ego can support self-expression, or become a barrier that resists growth and clings to illusion.
4. **Chitta (Memory and Subconscious Mind)** – *Chitta* stores impressions (*samskaras*), experiences and subconscious tendencies. It plays a central role in focus, meditation and deep thinking. In Yogic thought, *Chitta* is always in motion, undergoing fluctuations known as *Chitta Vrittis, or* mental modifications that shape how we perceive reality. These fluctuations create a veil, preventing us from experiencing pure awareness (*Satya*).

When these four elements – *Manas, Buddhi, Ahamkara* and *Chitta* – work in harmony, they support mental clarity, emotional balance and a deeper sense of inner peace. But when imbalanced, they give rise to various psychological and physical disturbances.

An overactive *Manas* may lead to anxiety and overthinking. A dominant *Ahamkara* may cause pride and conflict. A restless *Chitta* creates distractions and mental clutter. A weakened *Buddhi* results in poor decision-making. These imbalances create *Adhis* (mental stress) which, if unaddressed, manifest as *Vyadhis* (physical disease). True healing begins by restoring balance in the mind, which in turn brings harmony to energy and body.

Bringing Balance: NLP, Yogic Philosophy and Inner Healing

Neuro-Linguistic Programming (NLP) helps shift internal patterns by transforming how we speak to ourselves. Since thoughts shape our reality, NLP breaks limiting beliefs, rewires negative mental loops and aligns the subconscious with conscious goals, bridging *Manas* and *Buddhi* in a meaningful way.

Yogic philosophy emphasises *Viveka* (discernment) and *Vairagya* (detachment), teaching us to observe thoughts without being ruled by them. The aim of yogic practice is to help us transcend the fluctuations of the mind and access a deeper, clearer truth.

Inner Child Healing addresses emotional wounds rooted in early experiences. These often drive our survival-based responses, long after the original threat has passed. Healing the inner child builds emotional resilience, enabling us to respond rather than react, and to live from a space of self-awareness rather than fear.

By integrating tools like NLP, yogic wisdom, and inner healing, we create space for deep transformation – a transformation that aligns the mind, body and emotions, and supports long-term well-being.

Rewiring the Mind with NLP

"NLP is the bridge between where we are and where we want to be," says Magical Rafi, Founder and Director of Magic of Change and a world-renowned NLP trainer who introduced me to the magic of mind healing.

Throughout this book, one truth becomes clear: Our choices determine whether we move toward health or illness. But if we know this, why do we often make decisions that harm us?

The answer lies in the structure of the mind. Our values shape our identity. Identity forms beliefs. Beliefs drive our experiences and our experiences shape our personal reality. This reality, in turn, determines our habits and behaviours.

NLP techniques help us intervene at the belief level, where many self-sabotaging patterns begin. Our internal narratives, formed through past events, can either empower or limit us.

For example, repeating thoughts like "I'm always unwell" or "I can't handle stress" becomes a kind of instruction to the brain, reinforcing illness. NLP helps interrupt these thought loops and replace them with empowering alternatives such as "My body is always working to heal" or "I grow stronger each day." These new narratives reshape our brain's response, reduce stress and enhance healing.

Changing how we think changes how we feel, and how we heal.

Values – What We Hold Important in Life

Values act as an internal compass, shaping every choice we make. They're often unconscious, yet they steer our behaviour, day after day. Just like fingerprints, values are unique to each individual.

If you want real change in your lifestyle, your health or your happiness, it starts with getting clear about what truly matters to you.

Many patients I've worked with claimed to value health, yet their actions told a different story: skipped meals, no time for exercise and constant stress. Only when they paused to reflect – perhaps after a health scare or a moment of fatigue – did they realise that they had to align their actions with their values. Once they did, even small changes created a powerful momentum.

If you feel stuck, start by asking: What do I value most? Vitality? Peace? Balance? When your actions reflect your deepest values, life feels more meaningful, and healing becomes more sustainable.

Beliefs – What We Accept as True About Ourselves and the World

Our beliefs directly shape how we experience life. The *Pygmalion Effect* – where people live up to the expectations placed on them – demonstrates this clearly. A child who's told they're capable often performs better. An employee trusted by their manager takes more initiative. Beliefs have power.

In Naturopathy we trust the body's innate ability to heal. Every fever, wound or inflammation is part of this intelligent design. But if someone repeatedly believes 'My body is weak' or 'This illness is permanent', they create a mental and biochemical reality that resists healing.

Belief influences biology. Studies on the placebo effect show that when people expect recovery, the brain releases healing chemicals like dopamine and endorphins. The immune system activates, stress hormones reduce and healing accelerates.

Just as a teacher's belief can turn an average student into a star, our belief in the body's healing intelligence can awaken its full potential. Trust in your body. Speak to it with kindness. And believe in its remarkable power to restore balance.

So the next time doubt creeps in about your body's ability to heal and decide to succumb to disease, remember: Your body is listening to your thoughts. Choose those thoughts wisely.

Healing the Past: Inner Child Work

Many of us carry emotional wounds from childhood or even adulthood such as unresolved fears, neglect or limiting beliefs about not being 'good enough'. These deeply ingrained emotions don't just affect our thoughts; they also keep our nervous system in a prolonged state of stress, often without us realising it. To illustrate this, I'll share a few cases from my clinic.

Case 1: The Man Who Always Felt Alone

A man in his 60s came to me with anxiety and depression, both deeply rooted in a persistent feeling of loneliness. He said, *"Though I have a lovely family – three sons and a daughter – I always feel lonely. I don't know why."*

Over multiple sessions, we worked together to uncover the root cause. During a timeline regression, a vivid memory surfaced from when he was five years old. His parents had left him alone at home while they went to the hospital for the birth of his younger brother. Due to circumstances, they couldn't take him along.

The image of that moment was deeply imprinted in his subconscious mind; he clearly remembered watching them say goodbye, getting into the car and driving away. It was then that a belief was planted within him: **"I am alone in this world."**

Although his father returned within 20 minutes to take him along, the emotional imprint had already been made. He carried this subconscious wound throughout his life, shaping his emotional experiences and relationships. It wasn't until this session that he finally recognised, released and healed it.

Case 2: The Woman Who Feared the Seashore

I once worked with a 50-year-old woman who had travelled across the world's oceans with her sailor husband, yet she had an intense fear of standing near the seashore. She couldn't understand why.

During our session, I guided her through a timeline regression. She recalled an incident from when she was five years old. She had visited a beach with her parents when a huge wave suddenly swept her off her feet. Fortunately her parents caught her before she was carried away, but the terror of that moment remained imprinted in her subconscious.

Now, every time she stood on a beach and saw waves, her mind unconsciously triggered the same fear, as a protective mechanism. Though she had spent years travelling the oceans, her subconscious still linked the sight of waves to the terrifying childhood memory, preventing her from feeling safe on the shore.

Case 3: The Man Who Couldn't Complete Anything for Himself

Another man, one in his 40s, came to me complaining that he could never complete anything in his life. As I examined the pattern, I noticed that he was able to complete tasks for others, especially for people he loved, but struggled to do anything for himself.

Through memory analysis, he traced this behaviour back to a moment in childhood when his mother told him, "You are responsible for your three sisters; they are more important than you." Over time, this belief took root, shaping a pattern where he always prioritised others' needs over his own, sacrificing his desires. His subconscious mind had accepted this as a fundamental truth, making it nearly impossible for him to focus on himself without guilt or resistance.

These cases demonstrate the power of inner child work in uncovering and transforming hidden emotional imprints. In many situations, it is not our adult self that responds, but a younger, wounded version of us. Our subconscious mind records experiences in a way that logic and time cannot erase. By revisiting and healing the wounded inner child, we can replace limiting beliefs with self-compassion and emotional freedom. Once we understand where our pain originates, we create space for true healing and transformation.

The subconscious mind, influenced by the hippocampus (which governs memory) and the amygdala (which processes emotions), often triggers childhood-based reactions that may not be relevant to our present reality. Every response we have goes through a loop between these two centres. Imagine that you are coming to my clinic and waiting for a consultation. The moment you enter my room, your eyes take a picture of me and send it to your memory centre – the hippocampus – and ask, 'Have I seen him before?' Your hippocampus may say, 'I don't have an exact reference, but you have been with someone who looks similar.' Then your conscious brain takes this feedback to the emotional centre – the amygdala – to assess any emotional response. If you had a traumatic experience with someone who looks like me, your conscious brain might decide, 'Be careful with him.' As a result, you enter my room with an element of caution and fear, which in reality has nothing to do with me. No matter what I do, your reaction is already influenced by a past experience.

This subconscious loop affects how we perceive and respond to every situation in life, either positively or negatively. If it empowers us, it is beneficial. But if it limits us, we need to address it. I refer to these unresolved wounds as 'dark rooms' in our mind, hidden spaces that store past experiences and influence our present emotions and actions. If we do not address them, they continue to control our lives. This is where Inner Child Healing comes in.

Inner Child Healing is like cleaning out a long-forgotten room in our house filled with rotten potatoes; everyone subconsciously knows it's there, but they ignore it. However, true healing requires us to acknowledge and clear this space. It is important to note that memory is reconstructive – meaning that we do not store exact copies of past events, but rather reconstruct them based on current perceptions and emotions. Some fears are not always from direct experiences, but may be inherited through epigenetics or learned indirectly through observation.

The Five Steps of Inner Child Healing:

1. **Recognise that the room exists** – Acknowledge unresolved emotional wounds. Many times we may consciously forgive and even forget certain incidents, yet they continue to influence our behaviours and decisions. The first step is to recognise that our past experiences, even those buried deep in our

subconscious, may be governing, controlling and even manipulating us.

2. **Be willing to open the door** – Once acknowledged, facing these past experiences is often the hardest part. But it is essential. These wounds have been buried and decaying in our subconscious, manifesting in our daily lives through our behaviours and reactions. To truly heal, we must be willing to bring these hidden emotions to light and release them once and for all.
3. **Commit to the cleaning process** – This stage involves actively processing those emotions, analysing them rationally and reassuring our inner child that those fears, beliefs or traumas are no longer relevant. We need to remind ourselves that we have grown, matured, and are now fully equipped to handle life's challenges. Healing is not just about rationalisation; some traumas are stored in the body (somatic memory) and may require approaches like breath work, movement therapy or trauma-focussed techniques. There is no need to run from these emotions anymore – we are stronger than we think. If you don't feel strong right now, it's only because you haven't looked at the right parts of yourself. Shift your perspective, and you'll find your inner strength.
4. **Accept the mess along the way** – Just like cleaning a room, the process can get messy before it gets better. Revisiting painful memories can be uncomfortable, but it is a necessary part of healing. And once we get through it, we will experience an incredible sense of empowerment. We will begin to enjoy life with less emotional baggage weighing us down.
5. **Maintain a clean space** – Healing isn't just about clearing out old wounds; it's also about preventing new ones from accumulating. Now that we have understood the process, we must ensure that we no longer pile up unnecessary emotional burdens in our mind

space. Practicing emotional hygiene, setting healthy boundaries, and being mindful of our thoughts and reactions can help us maintain a balanced and peaceful inner world.

By working through these steps, we free ourselves from emotional baggage, allowing the body and mind to relax, heal and move forward with inner peace.

Mind healing modalities like NLP and Inner Child Healing empower individuals to take charge of their thoughts, emotions, and self-perception. By recognising and altering subconscious patterns, we pave the way for profound mental, emotional and physical transformation. When the mind heals, the body follows.

Bringing It All Together

Under the topic of *Mind*, I have detailed two approaches: activating the rest-and-heal mechanism and exploring mind-healing modalities to restore balance. You don't need to set aside hours each day to benefit from these practices; small, intentional shifts can make a big difference. Start your day with a few minutes of meditation, take deep breaths during stressful moments, laugh freely, connect with loved ones, note down happy moments and spend time in nature. Over time these simple habits retrain the nervous system, making relaxation and healing the default state rather than stress and survival.

The beauty of healing is that it empowers you to take charge of your well-being. By understanding and applying these techniques, you're not just managing symptoms, you're activating the body's deepest healing mechanisms. Healing isn't something that happens *to* us; it's something we create, moment by moment, through the choices we make. And the mind is where it all begins.

Each of these methods taps into the mind's ability to influence bodily functions, reinforcing the idea that healing is a holistic process where mental and emotional well-being directly impact physical health.

Embrace Rejection and Conquer Fear: The Path to Resilience and Growth

Rejection, when viewed through a constructive lens, becomes an invaluable teacher rather than a deterrent. It encourages growth, self-reflection and recalibration of goals. Those who face rejection often are the ones actively pursuing their aspirations, taking risks and pushing boundaries – hallmarks of meaningful achievement. Rejection strips away what isn't meant for us, guiding us toward opportunities better aligned with our purpose. It builds resilience by teaching us to weather discomfort and disappointment, strengthening our character and determination. Moreover, rejection invites us to reassess and refine our approach, helping us grow smarter and more strategic. Ultimately, rejection is not the end; it's a step in the redirection toward a life of deeper fulfilment and greater accomplishment. Those who embrace it as part of their journey cultivate a mindset that turns setbacks into stepping stones.

Fear is often a product of the mind, rooted in limiting beliefs and imagined outcomes that hold us back. It thrives on avoidance, growing stronger when left unchallenged. The antidote to fear is action – stepping into the unknown despite the discomfort. Each time you face what scares you, you reclaim a piece of your power, building courage and resilience. Over time, fear loses its grip, revealing that it was often an illusion. By confronting your fears, you expand your horizons, unlocking growth and the realisation that you are capable of far more than you believed. Transformation lies just beyond the edge of fear.

Fear is a limiting belief, which can be overcome by action; Do the things which scare you…until it won't!

Let me emphasise again – the human body possesses remarkable intelligence and inherently knows how to heal itself when given the right support. By integrating these techniques into daily life, we can guide the nervous system toward balance, fostering deep rest, repair and overall well-being. Healing isn't just about avoiding stress; it's about actively engaging in practices that restore and rejuvenate both body and mind. Through these natural and accessible methods, we don't just create change, we cultivate profound transformation, making true healing not just possible but inevitable.

CHAPTER 7

The Unseen

Microbiome: The Hidden World Within!

The Awakening

Just a few days after I joined the medical graduation course in Naturopathy and Yoga (BNYS), Dr Kavitha Venkidachalam stormed into our classroom. She's like that – she comes in with high energy that radiates everywhere she goes.

She was our lecturer for the first-year subject that introduced us to the basics of Naturopathy – PNC (Philosophy of Nature Cure) – along with other fundamental medical subjects like Anatomy, Physiology and Biochemistry.

Then she said something that shook us: "Germs don't cause disease!"

We, the students, looked at each other, confused. Were we in the wrong place? She was questioning one of the core beliefs of medical science!

Then she asked, "What causes diarrhoea?"

We answered, "House flies."

She continued, "Then why doesn't diarrhoea occur every time a housefly lands on food?"

We hesitated before replying, "Because it happens only if the fly carries germs."

She then asked, "What attracts house flies?"

We responded, "Rotten food, like a banana peel."

And then came her thought-provoking question:

"So what causes diarrhoea – the housefly, the germ or the banana peel?"

At that moment, she was introducing us to one of the fundamental concepts of Naturopathy: Germs are not the primary cause of disease; toxins are.

She went on to explain:

"Germs are opportunistic; they don't create disease out of nowhere. They only thrive where the conditions allow them to. If your body is clean and strong, germs can't harm you. But if your body is filled with accumulated toxins, it becomes a fertile ground for disease.

"Just as flies are drawn to decay, harmful microbes are more likely to thrive in a body burdened by waste and toxins. The real cause of disease isn't the germ – it's the environment that allows the germ to multiply. If the terrain is toxic, the germs flourish. If the terrain is clean, they can't."

That was an introduction to a new dimension of health, a universe - rather, a multiverse.

The multiverse of microbes.

From there on, we learned that what we had been taught about microbes and infections was only half-truth, or sometimes pure lies.

The Forgotten Microbial Majority

In the medical curriculum we have a dedicated subject for the study of pathogens: Microbiology. We are taught about disease-causing bacteria, viruses, fungi and parasites, and the all-out war we need to get into against these using disinfectants, vaccines and antibiotics. But here's the missing truth – these so-called 'pathogens' make up only a tiny fraction of the microbial world.

In reality, less than 1 percent of all microbes are harmful. The rest – the vast majority – are either harmless or beneficial, playing crucial roles in our health. Yet, this huge, life-sustaining microbial world goes unnoticed in our medical education for a long time.

We are raised to fear microbes, to see them as enemies, but the truth is, we live because of them. They digest our food, produce essential nutrients, regulate our immune system and even communicate with our brain. Without them, we wouldn't survive.

And yet, modern medicine's focus is on killing microbes – antibiotics, disinfectants, sterilisation – without realising that in doing so, we are weakening the very foundation of our health.

Dr Kavitha's words shattered our old beliefs and opened our eyes to a deeper truth: Health is not about fighting germs; it's about creating harmony in the internal environment. The body isn't a battlefield, it's an ecosystem. And just like any ecosystem, its well-being depends on balance, not war.

She left us with one final question: "If a garbage bin is filled with rotting food, would you blame the flies for the stench? Or would you clean the bin?"

And that, in one powerful analogy, she summed up the philosophy of Nature Cure.

Are We Fighting the Wrong Battle?

Microbes – commonly known as bacteria, viruses or fungi – often invoke fear in us. From childhood we're conditioned to see them as enemies, dangerous invaders threatening our health. We're taught to wage an unrelenting war against them.

Our daily routine reflects this battle. We start the day brushing our teeth, eliminating 99.9 percent of bacteria in our mouths. We bathe with antibacterial soaps, wiping out another 99.9 percent on our skin. We apply deodorants to kill odour-causing bacteria, eat off dishes scrubbed with germ-killing soap and walk on floors sanitised with chemical disinfectants. Even our curtains, wall paints and newspapers now boast antimicrobial properties. And just in case something survives, we finish the job with hand sanitisers. When illness strikes, we unleash our strongest weapon: antibiotics.

But is this battle truly worth winning?

Are microbes really so terrible that we must eliminate them indiscriminately? These microscopic beings are, in fact, our ancestors. They've existed for billions of years and have co-evolved with us.

Perhaps they deserve better understanding rather than blind extermination.

Let's imagine for a moment that our war against microbes is entirely successful. One fine day, all bacteria, viruses and fungi vanish. What happens then? Without microbes, organic matter wouldn't decompose properly. Nutrient cycles would collapse, soil fertility would plummet and the Earth would become a giant garbage dump. The entire biosphere would spiral into chaos. Without microbial life, plants would fail to thrive and the food chain would collapse.

Even the oxygen we breathe relies heavily on microbes like cyanobacteria, which produce a large share of atmospheric oxygen through photosynthesis. Without them, oxygen levels would steadily decline, putting all aerobic life at risk.

These consequences aren't just theoretical. The human body would be hit just as hard. Microbes in our gut break down food, produce vitamins and support immune function. Without them, digestion would falter, leading to malnutrition and disease.

They also help train our immune system, teaching it to recognise threats and avoid overreactions. Without that guidance, the immune system may become hypersensitive or underdeveloped, leading to a surge in allergies, autoimmune issues and vulnerability to new pathogens. Microbes even regulate energy metabolism, impacting our vitality in profound ways.

And now, it's time to rethink the much-discussed 'gut-brain connection' as the '*bacteria-brain connection*'. Beneficial bacteria influence mood, stress levels and cognition by producing neurotransmitters like serotonin. Without them, we may face increased anxiety, depression and neurological disorders.

Maybe we should be grateful that many of the products we use – like toothpaste, soaps and deodorants – don't fully deliver on their promise. If they truly eliminated 99.9 percent of microbes from our bodies, humanity might have vanished long ago.

Microbes and Host Behaviour: The Hidden Puppeteers

Microbes don't just live within us, they shape our world, often in ways we don't realise. For their survival, these microscopic organisms alter the environment they inhabit: the host body. When these changes benefit both the host and the microbes, we experience good health. But when they disrupt balance, we suffer, sometimes even facing illness or death. Below, we'll explore some fascinating instances where microbes manipulate their hosts, revealing just how deeply intertwined our lives are with these unseen forces.

1. The Zombie Ant: A Fungal Puppet Show

Deep in the rainforests, an unsuspecting carpenter ant goes about its day, unaware that a silent invader has taken hold. This invader is *Ophiocordyceps*, a parasitic fungus with a chilling mission: to control the ant's body and ensure its own survival.

Once inside, the fungus spreads, hijacking the ant's nervous system like a master puppeteer. At just the right moment, the infected ant is compelled to climb to a high point – a leaf or tree branch – where it locks its jaws in an eerie 'death grip'. There, the ant remains frozen as the fungus digests it from within, using its nutrients to fuel growth. Eventually, the fungus bursts from the ant's body, releasing spores into the air, ready to infect new hosts and continue its spine-chilling cycle of manipulation.

The ant, once a free creature, becomes nothing more than a vehicle for the fungus's survival. While this might seem like a horror story from the insect world, nature is full of such unsettling yet fascinating relationships.

2. Fearless Mice and the Cat's Deadly Embrace

Picture a mouse scurrying through the shadows, instinctively avoiding the scent of a cat. Normally, this fear is what keeps it alive. But when infected by *Toxoplasma gondii*, a microscopic parasite, something strange happens – the mouse loses its natural fear of cat odour. Instead, it begins to take reckless risks, wandering into dangerous territory.

Why? Because *Toxoplasma gondii* needs to enter a cat's body to complete its life cycle. By altering the mouse's behaviour, the parasite increases the likelihood of its host being eaten by a cat. Once inside, *T gondii* multiplies, is excreted in the cat's faeces and waits for another unsuspecting rodent to ingest it, continuing the cycle.

But here's where it gets even more intriguing – this parasite doesn't just affect rodents. Studies suggest that *T gondii* may influence human behaviour as well. Some researchers propose that infected individuals might exhibit changes in personality, increased risk-taking behaviour and even altered mental health. Could this parasite be subtly shaping human decisions in ways we don't yet fully understand? It's a chilling yet captivating thought.

3. The Rumen's Secret: How Cows Turn Grass into Energy

Not all microbe-host relationships are sinister. Some are vital partnerships that sustain life. A perfect example is the relationship between cows and their gut microbes.

Cows, like other ruminants, survive on a diet primarily composed of grass and fibrous plant material. But here's the catch – cows themselves lack the enzymes needed to break down cellulose, the tough fibre in plant cell walls. This is where their microbial partners come in.

Inside a cow's first stomach, or rumen, lives a complex community of bacteria, protozoa and fungi that work together to ferment and break down cellulose into usable energy. Microbes such as *Ruminococcus* and *Fibrobacter* produce enzymes that digest fibre, transforming it into fatty acids that the cow can absorb and use for energy. Additionally, some rumen bacteria synthesise essential vitamins like B12, which the cow cannot produce on its own.

Without these microbes, a cow wouldn't be able to extract enough nutrition from its plant-based diet to survive. In return, the microbes receive a warm, stable environment with a constant food supply. This perfect symbiosis showcases how microbes don't just manipulate their hosts, they can also form life-sustaining partnerships.

Microbes: The Silent Architects of Health

These examples offer a glimpse into how microbes have been shaping their hosts' behaviour for millions of years, sometimes to the host's detriment, sometimes for mutual benefit. From zombie ants and fearless mice to cows digesting grass, microbes are silent forces in nature. As microbiome research deepens, we're beginning to realise that their impact on human health, behaviour and decision-making may be greater than we ever imagined.

Microbes don't just live inside us; they can influence our actions, decisions and even emotions. While not all microbes are cunning manipulators, their influence reminds us of the deep interconnectedness of all life.

As we explore naturopathy and holistic healing, it's important to understand that our inner microbial world, gut flora, beneficial bacteria and even potential invaders play a key role in our health. Recognising these invisible allies allows us to better navigate our physical, mental and emotional well-being.

The next time you notice a sudden craving or shift in mood, it might just be a tiny microbial whisper at work.

The Overlooked 99 percent: The Microbial Guardians of Health

We often fear microbes, forgetting that we are more microbe than human – our bodies host trillions of them, outnumbering our own cells. These organisms are vital to the very life we strive to protect.

From birth, microbes shape our health in ways we barely acknowledge. They help digest food, produce essential vitamins, support immunity and influence mood. Our skin, mouth, gut and lungs are home to helpful bacteria working quietly to keep us healthy. Yet in our quest for cleanliness, we often destroy these allies with antibacterial products and harsh chemicals, unknowingly weakening our natural defences instead of strengthening them.

The Gut Microbiome: A Delicate Ecosystem

Of all the microbes that inhabit us, the gut microbiome is a powerhouse, central to digestion, immunity and mental health. Hosting trillions of bacteria, fungi and other organisms, it's like a rainforest ecosystem within us.

Beyond breaking down food, the gut microbiome plays a major role in keeping us healthy. When disrupted – due to poor diet, chronic stress, excessive antibiotics or toxins – its effects ripple throughout the body. One of the first signs is digestive distress. An imbalance in gut bacteria, or dysbiosis, can lead to bloating, IBS, constipation or inflammatory bowel disease. Harmful bacteria overpower the good, causing inflammation and immune overactivation.

And that's just the beginning. Since about 70 percent of our immune system resides in the gut, an unhealthy microbiome leaves us vulnerable to infections, allergies and chronic inflammation. A weakened gut barrier can allow harmful substances to leak into the bloodstream, triggering immune responses that contribute to long-term illness.

Most concerning is the link between poor gut health and autoimmune conditions. When microbial balance is lost, the immune system can become confused, attacking healthy cells. This has been linked to diseases like rheumatoid arthritis, multiple sclerosis and type 1 diabetes. Instead of defending us, the immune system turns inward, creating chronic inflammation and damage.

Understanding the gut's role reveals why its care is central to overall wellness. A balanced gut isn't just about digestion – it supports immunity, emotional resilience and disease prevention. When we nourish our gut, we nourish our whole being.

In Naturopathy there's a simple yet powerful truth: *"Gut health is the best health, and gut hygiene is the best hygiene."* It's a reminder that the path to well-being starts from within.

The First Dose of Life: Microbial Inheritance at Birth

Our journey with microbes begins at birth. When a baby is born through the vaginal canal, it receives its first microbial 'inoculation' – a vital dose of beneficial bacteria from the mother. Remarkably, during pregnancy, a woman's vaginal microbiome shifts to favour milk-digesting bacteria. Why? Because nature intended it that way. These microbes colonise the newborn's gut, preparing it to digest the first milk, or colostrum. Rich in fats and amino acids, colostrum feeds both the baby and the new bacteria, laying the foundation for a lifelong symbiotic relationship.

But what about babies born via C-section? They miss this first microbial gift. Without it, their gut is less prepared to process milk, making them more susceptible to digestive issues. Research shows that C-section babies often have a different microbiome makeup, linked to a higher risk of allergies, asthma and autoimmune conditions. Early microbial exposure is key to immune training, digestive function and reducing inflammation.

Missing this initial microbial inheritance can delay the development of a healthy microbiome, with possible long-term effects. Still, interventions like skin-to-skin contact, breastfeeding and, in some cases, microbiome seeding (swabbing the baby with vaginal fluids) can help close the gap and support a healthier start.

Microbes: The Immune System's First Teachers

Once inside the baby, these microbes begin their crucial task: training the immune system. At birth, this system is like an untrained army, unsure of how to tell friend from foe. Microbes act as instructors, teaching it what belongs and what doesn't, helping distinguish between harmless and harmful invaders.

This training is essential. If the immune system misidentifies friendly microbes, it can overreact, causing allergies. If it's too aggressive, it may attack the body's own cells, leading to autoimmune diseases. If undertrained, it might not respond to real threats, leaving the body open to infections.

Microbes mediate this process. They stimulate immune cells and encourage tolerance toward good bacteria while identifying pathogens. They also promote the growth of regulatory T-cells, which keep the immune response balanced and prevent excessive inflammation. Without microbial guidance, the immune system may misfire, contributing to chronic inflammation and disease.

Microbes and Skin Health

Your skin isn't just a barrier; it's a vibrant ecosystem full of microbes. These beneficial organisms maintain skin health, fend off pathogens and control inflammation. They create a competitive environment, where helpful bacteria keep harmful ones in check, preventing infections and skin disorders.

One fascinating group is ammonia-oxidising bacteria (AOB). These microbes break down sweat into beneficial compounds that balance skin pH and reduce body odour naturally. Rather than relying on chemical-heavy deodorants and skincare products, a healthy microbiome can keep your skin fresh and balanced.

Disrupting the skin's microbiome through harsh soaps, antibiotics or toxins can lead to acne, eczema and premature ageing. Some microbes also produce natural moisturisers and aid in wound healing. Supporting this microbial balance with gentle skincare and minimal chemical exposure promotes vibrant, resilient skin.

Microbes and Gut Integrity

Picture your gut as a tightly secured compound with a selective entry system. Microvilli act as gates, absorbing nutrients while blocking harmful substances. *(Microvilli are tiny, finger-like projections lining the intestinal wall that increase surface area for absorption and serve as a selective barrier.)* Beneficial microbes are the guards, ensuring this system works smoothly.

The 'cement' holding this structure together is made of short-chain fatty acids (SCFAs), produced when gut bacteria ferment fibre from food. SCFAs help seal the gut lining, reduce inflammation and maintain a strong barrier. When this system is intact, essential nutrients are absorbed and invaders are kept out.

But when beneficial microbes decline, SCFA production drops and the gut lining weakens, creating gaps. This condition, often called leaky gut syndrome, lets toxins, undigested food and pathogens leak into the bloodstream. The immune system reacts, sparking inflammation, allergies and even autoimmunity.

Leaky gut has been linked to digestive issues, skin problems, mental health struggles and metabolic disorders. By feeding gut microbes with fibre-rich foods, prebiotics and probiotics, we can rebuild this barrier and restore balance, supporting overall resilience and well-being.

Microbes and Energy Production

Surprisingly, microbes contribute to our energy levels in ways we often overlook. Certain gut bacteria help break down food, assist in nutrient metabolism and even influence mitochondrial function. The gut microbiome also affects blood sugar regulation, helping to prevent fatigue and metabolic issues.

Ever noticed unexpected weight gain after pregnancy, antibiotics, or hospitalisation, even without dietary changes? That's because it's not just what you eat, but who's digesting it. Changes in gut bacteria can influence how many calories you extract from food. Some microbes are more efficient at pulling energy from food, leading to increased calorie absorption.

This is why gut diversity matters. Like a thriving forest compared to a monoculture, a diverse microbiome helps maintain metabolic balance. Eating a wide range of fibre-rich, fermented and whole foods nourishes various microbial species, supporting steady energy and overall vitality.

Microbes and Neurotransmitters

Ever wondered why your mood feels off even when life seems fine? The answer might lie in your gut. The brain and gut are constantly communicating via the gut-brain axis, with microbes playing a central role.

These microbes don't just aid digestion, they produce neurotransmitters that affect mood, stress and focus. About 90 percent of serotonin, the 'happiness chemical', is made in the gut. Dopamine, linked to motivation, and GABA, which helps you feel calm, are also produced by gut bacteria.

When your gut microbiome is imbalanced – too many harmful bacteria, not enough beneficial ones – neurotransmitter production suffers. This can contribute to anxiety, depression and brain fog.

So if you feel constantly stressed or struggle with focus and mood swings, your gut health might be influencing your brain more than you realise. Taking care of your microbes means taking care of your mind.

Rethinking Our Relationship with Microbes

We are more than just human; we are living ecosystems. Our health depends on the trillions of microbes we host. In fact, microbial cells outnumber human cells and play key roles in digestion, immunity, metabolism and mental health. When their balance is disrupted – a state called dysbiosis – our risk of inflammation and disease rises.

Humans often see the world in black and white, good or bad. But microbes aren't inherently either. Their behaviour reflects the environment we create. Our diet, stress levels and exposure to toxins shape our microbial ecosystem. Instead of viewing microbes as enemies or allies, it's more accurate to see them as responsive, adaptive life forms. When conditions are right, they promote health. When disturbed, they can contribute to disease.

The Role of Food in Shaping Our Microbial World

Food is one of the most powerful tools for shaping our microbiome. Every meal influences which microbes thrive or fade. What we eat fuels not just us, but also our gut's microbial residents.

Take sugar, for instance. Refined sugars and processed carbs feed microbes that thrive on fast energy. These sugar-loving bacteria shift the gut environment in ways that can harm microbial balance. Our gut naturally supports anaerobic microbes like *Bifidobacteria* and *Lactobacilli*. But high sugar intake can favour oxygen-tolerant species, reducing microbial diversity and increasing inflammation.

Sugar fermentation also produces excess lactic acid and other by-products that can irritate the gut lining, contributing to leaky gut syndrome. This allows harmful substances into the bloodstream, triggering systemic inflammation and potentially worsening autoimmune, metabolic and cardiovascular disorders.

The Power of Fibre: Supporting Beneficial Microbes

Unlike sugar, dietary fibre has the opposite effect – it fuels beneficial microbes. Since fibre can't be digested by human enzymes, it reaches the colon intact, where gut bacteria ferment it into compounds that support health.

One key role of fibre is preserving the gut's anaerobic environment. As microbes ferment fibre, they consume oxygen, helping maintain the low-oxygen conditions in which beneficial bacteria thrive. This supports a balanced and resilient microbial ecosystem.

Fibre fermentation also produces short-chain fatty acids (SCFAs) like butyrate, acetate and propionate. These nourish the gut lining, strengthen the intestinal barrier and reduce inflammation. Butyrate, in particular, is crucial for gut integrity, immune regulation and even brain function. Research shows SCFAs can support mental health by influencing neurotransmitter levels, helping reduce anxiety and depression.

Over time, a fibre-rich diet offers lasting benefits. Populations with high fibre intake show lower rates of obesity, autoimmune conditions and digestive issues. By choosing whole, fibre-rich foods, we promote microbial diversity while naturally keeping harmful bacteria in check.

Nourishing the Microbiome: Prebiotics and Probiotics

Supporting our gut microbiome means focussing on both prebiotics - foods that feed good bacteria and probiotics - foods that contain live beneficial microbes that help restore balance.

Prebiotics are special fibres and plant compounds that nourish helpful bacteria, allowing them to flourish. Found in foods like bananas, apples, onions, garlic, leeks, asparagus, oats, barley, lentils and nuts like flaxseeds and chia, these fibres travel to the colon, where they fuel the production of SCFAs and encourage a healthy gut environment.

Probiotics, in contrast, are live bacteria that replenish microbial populations, especially after disruptions like antibiotics, stress or poor diet. Probiotic-rich foods include fermented dairy like yogurt and kefir, fermented vegetables such as sauerkraut and kimchi, and traditional drinks like kombucha and *kanji*. These introduce beneficial bacteria that aid digestion, boost immunity and support gut barrier health.

By choosing foods that nourish our microbiome, we create an inner ecosystem geared toward balance and vitality. Microbes aren't fixed; they respond to the conditions we provide. Daily choices – what we eat, how we handle stress and our environment – shape this internal world. Instead of labelling microbes as good or bad, we should understand that their actions depend on the conditions we create. Cultivating a diverse, balanced microbiome is a powerful step toward long-term health and resilience.

Understanding Soluble Fibre and Resistant Starch

Soluble fibre and resistant starch are two powerful nutrients that can transform your gut health. They aid digestion, stabilise blood sugar and nourish beneficial gut bacteria. Soluble fibre dissolves in water, forming a gel-like substance that slows digestion and regulates glucose absorption. It also gets fermented by gut bacteria, producing short-chain fatty acids (SCFAs) like butyrate, which strengthens the gut lining, lowers inflammation and supports immunity. Great sources of soluble fibre include oats, flaxseeds, beans, lentils, apples and psyllium husk. Less-known but excellent options include ladies' finger (okra), which has soothing mucilage for gut protection, and passion fruit, rich in pectin that feeds beneficial microbes.

Resistant starch functions differently. Unlike regular starch, it escapes digestion in the small intestine and reaches the colon intact, where it becomes food for good bacteria. These microbes produce SCFAs, especially butyrate, reinforcing the gut lining and preventing issues like leaky gut. Resistant starch also enhances insulin sensitivity, helping with blood sugar control. You can find it in green bananas, cooked-and-cooled potatoes or rice, legumes and whole grains. Raw jackfruit is an outstanding source, rich in resistant starch and perfect for blood sugar and gut health.

Some foods are especially gut-friendly because they offer both soluble fibre and resistant starch. Raw jackfruit is one such natural prebiotic; it feeds beneficial bacteria, supports butyrate production and stabilises blood sugar. Okra is another, thanks to its gut-soothing mucilage. Guava is high in fibre, boosts gut motility and the seeds act as a natural gut cleanser. Passion fruit, with its rich pectin content, aids digestion, reduces bloating and supports beneficial microbes.

Eating more soluble fibre and resistant starch doesn't just benefit digestion, it also helps balance your gut bacteria, improve metabolism, reduce inflammation and strengthen your gut barrier. A healthy gut can even help regulate hormones, as microbes play a key role in producing neurotransmitters and hormones.

By adding more fibre-rich foods like raw jackfruit, okra, guava and passion fruit to your meals, you can naturally support digestion, boost immunity and enhance overall gut health. Small dietary shifts toward whole, fibre-dense foods can lead to lasting health improvements and reinforce a gut-friendly lifestyle.

Stress, Relaxation and the Hidden World of Microbes

We usually think of stress as a mental or emotional burden – tight deadlines, conflicts or feeling overwhelmed. But stress also impacts the trillions of microbes living in your gut. These organisms aren't just bystanders; they respond to emotions and influence digestion, immunity and inflammation. Chronic stress disrupts this microbial community, making the body more vulnerable to disease.

When stress hormones like cortisol, adrenaline and norepinephrine surge, they suppress beneficial bacteria like *Lactobacilli* and *Bifidobacteria*, causing imbalances (dysbiosis). This can trigger digestive problems and inflammation, and lower immunity. Over time, stress also weakens the gut lining, allowing toxins to escape into the bloodstream – a condition often referred to as 'leaky gut'.

Relaxation: The Key to a Healthy Gut Microbiome

When you're relaxed, your gut microbiome begins to thrive again. Lower cortisol levels allow beneficial microbes like *Bifidobacteria* and *Lactobacilli* to repopulate, restoring balance. This helps improve digestion, reduce bloating and support immune strength. Relaxation also helps repair the gut lining, keeping harmful substances out of your bloodstream.

Your gut is shaped not just by your diet but also by how you feel. Chronic stress weakens the gut barrier, disrupts microbial balance and fuels inflammation. The good news? Relaxation is a powerful way to reverse that process. It can restore balance, ease digestion and reduce inflammation.

Making space for relaxation through practices like deep breathing, meditation, quality sleep or spending time in nature does more than calm your mind. It creates a healthy inner ecosystem that supports long-term health, resilience and well-being.

Reconnecting with Nature: Restoring Our Microbial Balance

How do we rebuild our lost microbial diversity? The answer is simple: reconnect with nature. Walking barefoot on grass – known as earthing – introduces beneficial microbes into our system while also grounding our body's electrical charge, reducing stress and inflammation. Gardening, touching soil and spending time in green spaces can also reintroduce friendly microbes. Even hugging or shaking hands allows microbial exchange that strengthens our immune system. Interestingly, soil bacteria like *Mycobacterium vaccae* have been shown to boost serotonin, the feel-good chemical in the brain. This may explain why we feel calm and uplifted after time in nature.

From a naturopathic lens, nature is not just a backdrop, it's vital to healing. The more we interact with the natural world, the more we align with our biological blueprint. Our ancestors lived in harmony with nature, constantly exposed to microbes that kept them resilient. Small lifestyle changes - spending more time outdoors, touching the earth, eating unprocessed foods and reducing our obsession with sterilisation - can help restore microbial balance. In doing so, we support not just gut health, but the body's innate ability to heal and thrive.

Superbugs: When Antibiotics Fight Back

For decades, antibiotics have been a medical miracle, saving countless lives from infections once considered deadly. A cut, sore throat, or lung infection that could have turned fatal a century ago became easy to treat with a simple pill. It felt like bacteria had been conquered.

But now, that very solution is becoming a problem. Bacteria are smart and incredibly adaptable. When we take antibiotics, it's like dropping a bomb - they kill harmful and beneficial bacteria alike. The survivors evolve, becoming resistant to the drugs. These bacteria come back stronger, passing on their resistance, forming what we now call 'superbugs'. You've heard the phrase 'What doesn't kill you makes you stronger'. That's exactly what happens with bacteria. Over time, these superbugs become resistant to multiple antibiotics, creating a crisis known as antimicrobial resistance (AMR) - a growing global threat. Infections that were once easily treatable, like pneumonia or UTIs, are now tougher to manage. In some cases, doctors are left with no effective treatment. We could face a future where routine surgeries or a small cut could lead to life-threatening infections, much like in the pre-antibiotic era.

How did we get here? Misuse and overuse of antibiotics are a major part of the problem. People often take them for viral illnesses like colds or flu, despite antibiotics only working on bacteria. In agriculture, antibiotics are used to prevent disease and boost growth in animals, creating resistant strains that enter our food and environment. Even our soaps, sprays and sanitisers are packed with antimicrobials, contributing to resistance.

This overuse disrupts our natural microbial balance. Instead of blasting our microbiome at the first sign of illness, we need to support our body's innate defence systems. It's not about declaring war on all bacteria; it's about managing the 1 percent that cause disease more strategically. This is in line with Naturopathy's Soil-Seed Theory, which teaches that disease arises not just from harmful microbes (the 'seeds'), but from the internal state of the body (the 'soil') they grow in. The healthier our internal terrain, the harder it is for disease to take root.

The Infamous 1 percent: Villains or Scapegoats?

So far, we've explored the 99 percent, the vast majority of microbes that quietly support our health, aid digestion and strengthen our immunity. But no story is complete without mentioning the remaining 1 percent, the ones we've been taught to fear. These are the so-called villains, the pathogens that make headlines, spark outbreaks and create a sense of panic and helplessness. *Salmonella* causes food poisoning, *Mycobacterium tuberculosis* leads to tuberculosis and *Vibrio cholerae* is responsible for deadly cholera outbreaks. These bacteria have been portrayed as relentless enemies, lurking in our food and water, and even within us, waiting to strike.

The message we've grown up with is clear: "The enemy is already inside the fort and our internal army has failed. The only way to survive is to hire a private army from outside and wait for fate to decide." This mindset has fuelled an aggressive approach - overuse of antibiotics, excessive sterilisation and an all-out war against microbes. But has this truly made us healthier? Or have we weakened our natural defences in the process?

As a naturopath, my answer is simple: focus on your strength, not on your enemies. Instead of obsessing over eradicating harmful bacteria, strengthen your body's resilience. A strong immune system, a balanced microbiome and a healthy internal environment make it difficult for pathogens to take hold. Rather than fearing the 1 percent, we should ask, "Why do they thrive in some and not in others?" The real solution lies not in destruction but in restoration, not in fear but in balance.

Our approach is based on Soil-Seed Theory - a beautiful concept that Dr Kavitha explained to me when I was a student, which I mentioned at the beginning of this chapter. To delve deep into this we need to know, how do we get infections?

How Do We Get Infections?

It's well established that our lifestyle plays a key role in the development of metabolic diseases, often referred to as non-communicable diseases. But what about infectious diseases? We know that the primary culprits behind these are microbes or pathogens, commonly called agents. The general belief is that these agents attack us, making us sick, and that we're helpless in fighting them off without medicines or vaccines. While our body's immune system does play a role in preventing and fighting infections, many of us are taught to believe that it isn't sufficient on its own. This leads to the assumption that infections automatically mean we need medicines. But how true is this?

While the presence of a pathogen is necessary for an infectious disease to occur, it cannot act alone. For a disease to develop, two other factors must contribute equally. This concept is explained by the triad of infectious diseases, which includes the agent (pathogen), the host (our body) and the environment. These three factors work together to determine whether an infection occurs. If even one of these factors doesn't contribute, the disease cannot develop.

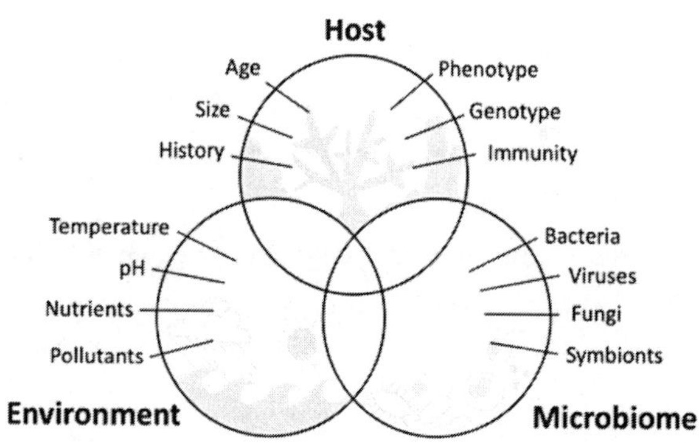

Understanding this triad gives us a clearer picture of how infections happen. It's not just about a microbe attacking us; it's about how our body responds and how the environment influences the interaction. Let's delve into the triad of infectious diseases to clarify this further:

The Agent: More than Just a Germ

When we hear about infectious diseases, the first thought that comes to mind is usually the pathogen itself - the bacteria, virus, fungus or parasite responsible for the illness. It's true that these microscopic organisms are necessary for an infection to occur, but simply coming into contact with them doesn't mean we'll automatically fall ill. Whether or not a pathogen actually causes disease depends on several factors, including how strong and aggressive it is, how much of it enters the body and how well it can evade the body's defences.

Some microbes are naturally more virulent, meaning they have powerful mechanisms to invade and damage the body. For example, the bacteria *Mycobacterium tuberculosis* can survive inside immune cells, making it difficult for the body to eliminate it. Others, like *Salmonella*, can produce toxins that cause food poisoning. But even the most dangerous pathogens need a sufficient dose to cause illness. A few viral particles may not be enough to overwhelm the immune system, whereas a large exposure - such as inhaling a high concentration of flu virus in a closed space - makes infection more likely.

Another key factor is the pathogen's ability to evade the body's defences. Some bacteria, like *Helicobacter pylori* (linked to stomach ulcers), can survive stomach acid, while certain viruses, like HIV, directly attack the immune system itself. However, the presence of a pathogen alone does not determine whether a person gets sick; it's the interaction between the microbe, the immune system and the overall health of the body that truly matters.

The Host: More than Just Immunity

Approximately 40 percent of the Indian population harbours *Mycobacterium tuberculosis*, but in its latent form, known as Latent Tuberculosis Infection (LTBI). However, only 5–10 percent of these individuals may develop active tuberculosis (TB) in their lifetime.

Why doesn't everyone with the bacteria develop the disease?

This is because the transition from latent to active TB isn't determined by the bacteria alone, but by the health of the host. When it comes to infections, we often focus on the pathogen as the primary culprit, but the real question is: Why do some people fall ill, while others, despite being exposed to the same microbe, remain perfectly fine?

The answer lies in the condition of the host. The body isn't just a passive battleground for infections; it is an intelligent, dynamic system capable of defending itself, adapting and even healing when given the right support.

Your immunity is the major factor that decides this. A strong immune system can detect and neutralise invaders before they cause harm. But immunity isn't just about having enough white blood cells or antibodies; it is deeply influenced by lifestyle, nutrition, stress levels and overall vitality. A body nourished with wholesome, natural foods and supported by restorative sleep and regular movement is far more resistant to infections. However, physical health alone doesn't tell the full story.

The mind also plays a crucial role. Emotions, thoughts and beliefs shape how the body responds to threats. Chronic stress, anxiety and fear suppress immune function, making the body more vulnerable to infections. On the other hand, a positive mind-set, emotional balance and a deep connection with the body's signals enhance resilience. This is why people who practice mindfulness, meditation and relaxation techniques often experience fewer illnesses and recover faster when they do fall ill. The body and mind work together as a unified system - when one is strong, the other follows. True resistance to disease isn't just about killing germs; it's about creating an internal environment where health naturally thrives, making the body an unsuitable place for disease to take hold.

The Environment: A Silent Influencer

When we think about infections, we often focus on the germs themselves or the body's ability to fight them. But there's another crucial player in this equation: the environment. The world around us can either help or hinder the spread of disease, acting as a silent influencer in how pathogens survive, thrive or fade away.

Physical factors such as temperature, humidity and sanitation play a major role in determining whether a pathogen can survive long enough to infect someone. Some bacteria and viruses thrive in warm, moist conditions, while others prefer cooler, drier environments. Poor sanitation creates breeding grounds for harmful microbes, allowing diseases to spread more easily. A simple example is cholera, which thrives in contaminated water, making proper sanitation and clean drinking water essential in preventing outbreaks.

Beyond physical conditions, social factors also shape the way diseases spread. In densely populated areas, infections can travel rapidly from person to person, as seen in cities where close human contact makes it easier for airborne viruses to spread. Access to healthcare also plays a significant role - people with timely medical care and good hygiene practices are far less likely to suffer severe infections or pass them on to others. Cultural habits, like handshaking or communal dining, can influence exposure to germs, sometimes increasing the risk of transmission without people even realising it.

On a larger scale, ecological balance determines how frequently humans come into contact with new and potentially dangerous microbes. Activities like deforestation, urban expansion and wildlife trade disturb natural ecosystems, bringing humans closer to animals that may carry unfamiliar pathogens. Many of the most dangerous viral outbreaks in recent history - such as Ebola, SARS and COVID 19 - have been linked to viruses jumping from animals to humans due to environmental disruptions. When we alter nature, we unknowingly create pathways for new diseases to emerge.

Understanding the role of the environment in disease spread helps us see that health isn't just about individual choices; it's also about the world we live in.

What Are We Doing Conventionally?

Conventional medical approaches primarily focus on controlling the **agent** - such as using vaccines to prevent infections, or antibiotics and antivirals to eliminate pathogens. Additionally, significant efforts are directed toward modifying the **environment** through measures like improving sanitation, promoting hygiene or implementing strategies such as social distancing. These methods are undoubtedly effective in reducing the spread and impact of infectious diseases.

However, one critical element of the triad - the **host** - often receives less attention in these strategies. The host's condition, including immunity, mental resilience and adaptability, is a vital factor in determining susceptibility to infections. Yet, conventional approaches seldom emphasise strengthening the host's internal defences, such as fostering a healthy lifestyle, enhancing nutrition, managing stress or addressing emotional and psychological well-being. By focussing primarily on external factors, conventional methods may overlook the host's natural ability to resist and recover from infections, which is crucial for long-term health and resilience.

Because of this, humanity finds itself in a constant state of vulnerability to infections. At any moment, a new infection can emerge, triggering widespread fear and anxiety. In response, we pour immense effort and resources into developing drugs or vaccines specific to the new threat, and after a long battle we momentarily breathe a sigh of relief - only for the next infection to surface.

This cycle has become a never-ending tragedy, where we are perpetually at war, trying to create agent-specific weapons for each new pathogen. This reactive approach leaves us in a continuous state of defence, chasing after emerging threats instead of addressing the root causes that make us susceptible. It's a reminder that true resilience lies not just in fighting pathogens but in strengthening the host - our bodies and minds - to reduce the very conditions that allow infections to thrive.

The Soil and Seed Theory: Cultivating Health from Within

Is there an alternative approach to this cycle, which has already proven to be ineffective in the long run? Can we adopt a better strategy to manage infections more sustainably and effectively?

The answer lies in the Soil and Seed Theory, a fundamental concept in Naturopathy.

Imagine that you are trying to grow crops. If the soil is poor, lacking nutrients and full of weeds, even the best seeds won't grow properly. On the other hand, if the soil is rich, well-nourished and balanced, healthy crops will flourish, while weeds struggle to survive. Our body works the same way. The 'soil' represents our internal environment - our immune system, gut health and overall vitality. The 'seeds' are the pathogens (bacteria, viruses, fungi) that attempt to take root. If the body is strong and balanced, harmful microbes struggle to thrive, and the risk of illness is significantly reduced.

Rather than focussing on killing every potential pathogen, the key to long-term health is improving the quality of the soil - our body's ability to resist, recover and thrive. A body that is well-nourished, well-rested and emotionally balanced does not provide a fertile ground for infections. Instead of fighting the same battles repeatedly, wouldn't it make more sense to strengthen our natural defences so that disease has no chance to take hold in the first place?

The Body's Natural Power: A Built-In Defence System

Our bodies are not helpless victims waiting to be attacked by diseases. We are equipped with an incredible self-defence system that is designed to protect, repair and heal. The immune system acts like a personal security force, recognising and eliminating harmful invaders before they can cause harm. But this defence system isn't just about white blood cells and antibodies; our body's natural healing mechanisms are constantly at work, repairing tissues, regenerating cells and restoring balance after injury or illness.

A major player in this process is the gut microbiome - a diverse community of beneficial bacteria that not only helps with digestion but also strengthens immunity, regulates inflammation and even affects mental well-being. A well-balanced microbiome creates an internal environment where harmful microbes struggle to survive. Instead of fearing microbes and trying to eliminate them all, the real key to health is maintaining a strong internal ecosystem where good bacteria thrive and naturally keep harmful ones in check.

A Shift from Fear to Empowerment

The Soil and Seed Theory is a wake-up call, a reminder that health isn't about constantly fighting external threats. Instead of living in fear of germs, we should focus on strengthening our own body so that it naturally resists disease. The stronger our soil, the less chance harmful seeds have to take root.

So, the real question is, are we going to continue relying on external interventions, or are we ready to take responsibility for our health and cultivate a body that thrives naturally? The choice is ours. When we work with nature instead of against it, true health isn't just possible; it becomes effortless.

Fighting Infections Naturally: Winning the Internal Battle

All the strategies we discussed - building a strong immune system, maintaining gut health and leading a balanced lifestyle - work well in times of peace, when our body is not under attack. But what happens when we are already at war, when an infection has taken hold? Do we switch to all-out attack mode, bombarding the body with external treatments? Or do we continue strengthening our natural defences?

The answer in Naturopathy is clear: never weaken your army, never support the enemy. The moment an infection sets in, the focus should be on cutting off the pathogen's supply lines and making the body an inhospitable place for it to survive.

Pathogens, especially bacteria and fungi, thrive on certain nutrients, particularly sugar. When we continue consuming sugary foods, refined carbohydrates and processed junk, we are unknowingly feeding the very microbes that are causing illness. Instead of strengthening the body, we end up strengthening the disease. The first step, therefore, is to stop feeding the infection.

One of the most effective ways to fight an infection naturally is to switch to a naturopathic elimination diet or fasting. Fasting is not about depriving the body, but about giving it the time and space it needs to heal. When we stop feeding the pathogens, the body can redirect its energy towards recovery.

This also activates a powerful natural process called autophagy, or 'self-eating', where the body begins to break down and recycle damaged cells, dead pathogens and unwanted foreign invaders. This process cleans up the battlefield, strengthens immunity and accelerates healing.

However, fasting and elimination diets should be done under proper guidance, especially when the body is fighting an active infection. A Naturopathy or Yoga physician can help you choose the best approach for your body's needs, ensuring that you heal safely and effectively.

When illness strikes, many people panic and start looking for quick fixes, often turning to strong medications that suppress symptoms rather than support healing. While emergency medicine has its place, true healing comes from within. Instead of waging war on our body with excessive treatments, we should support our natural defences and trust the body's innate wisdom to restore balance.

The goal is not just to survive an infection, but to emerge stronger. And that happens when we work with nature, not against it.

CHAPTER 8
The Facilitator

Elements: The Cosmos You Are!

In Kerala, India, we don't really have four seasons, like in some parts of the world.

Instead, the year can be split in two: blazing summer and pouring rain.

From December through May, Kerala is warm and humid, with the sun beaming for most of the day. The heat peaks around midday, making the air feel heavy, as summer builds toward May. Yet, thanks to Kerala's closeness to the Arabian Sea, we're spared severe heatwaves. The coastal breeze brings relief, and though rivers shrink under the sun, the land patiently awaits the life-giving rains.

Then, right on cue, June 1st arrives, and everything shifts. The sky darkens, the winds rise and suddenly, the skies burst open. The monsoon has arrived. It doesn't drizzle, it pours. Torrential rain sweeps away the heat and dust, and the scent of wet earth fills the air.

For months we live by the rhythm of rain. First comes the southwest monsoon, soaking everything. Then, by October, the northeast monsoon follows, its rains gentler but often paired with evening thunder. By late November, the cycle is ready to begin again.

The first showers always bring relief, but also concern. The cool rain refreshes body and mind, yet it invites infections. Ironically, this is also when schools reopen after two months of vacation. Parents, already anxious about school, now worry about keeping their kids dry and healthy.

While most children watch the rain from behind closed windows, our daughters, Bhadra and Devi, are outside, laughing and getting drenched. Unlike most parents in our neighbourhood who rush to keep their kids indoors, my wife, Dr Lakshmi Nair, and I, both naturopaths, do the opposite.

We send them out.

Because we believe nature heals. Kerala, God's Own Country, is filled with natural beauty, and the rain isn't just water, it's life, energy and renewal. The soil beneath our feet isn't just mud, it's medicine. It's meant to be felt, embraced and enjoyed. So while others hide from it, our family dances in it, believing that sometimes the best way to stay healthy is to trust nature.

The Five Elements: Aligning with Nature for Balance

Ancient traditions recognised that everything in existence, including our bodies, is composed of five fundamental elements: Earth, Water, Fire, Air and Ether. Just as nature thrives through the balance of these elements, our well-being depends on remaining aligned with them. This practice, known as *Panchamahabhootha Upasana*, offers a powerful way to restore harmony in both mind and body.

Our connection to these elements is not just philosophical, it's deeply physical. Earth forms the foundation of our being, shaping our muscles, bones and tissues. Just as soil nourishes plants, the food we eat, grown from the earth, replenishes our strength and resilience. Water flows through us as blood, lymph and fluids, mirroring the rivers and oceans that sustain life. It delivers oxygen and nutrients to our cells, cleansing and hydrating us, just as rain refreshes the land.

Fire is the force behind transformation. In the body, it manifests as digestion, metabolism and cellular activity, just as the sun fuels life on Earth. When balanced, this internal fire gives us vitality; when disturbed, it affects our health and energy. Air is the breath of life, the force that moves within and around us. It flows through our lungs, circulates in our blood and sustains every cell. The air we breathe influences our well-being directly, and conscious breathing helps calm the mind and energise the body.

Then there is Ether, the most subtle yet profound element. It's the space that allows everything to exist, the openness within and around us. It's found in the stillness between breaths, the silence of deep thought and the vast sky above. Connecting to this space - through meditation, stillness or simply observing nature - awakens a deeper awareness of self and the world. Ether is often associated with energy in all forms and, in spiritual traditions, with the soul. Called *Akasha* in Sanskrit, it is seen as the medium of consciousness, the bridge between the physical and the divine.

These five elements are not just within us; they shape the world we live in. The Earth beneath our feet, the mountains and the nourishing soil mirror the structure and stability within our bodies. The rivers and rain that flow through nature sustain us as water flows through our veins. The sun that energises life reflects our inner fire. The air shared by all beings moves through forests, cities and oceans, just as it flows within us. And Ether - the space through which birds soar, trees grow and the universe expands - is the same vast presence within, giving rise to thought, awareness and consciousness.

Scientific research confirms what ancient wisdom taught: Immersing ourselves in nature-rich environments improves both physical and mental well-being. Studies show biodiverse ecosystems offer greater psychological benefits than monoculture green spaces, fostering deeper restoration and connection. Forest bathing, for instance, is proven to reduce stress hormones, lower blood pressure and enhance cognitive clarity. Mere virtual exposure to nature has been shown to uplift mood and focus, proving that even indirect connections can promote healing.

When we immerse ourselves in nature, we don't just observe the elements, we reconnect with them. Walking barefoot strengthens our foundation, drinking pure water rehydrates and renews, breathing fresh air revitalises, and basking in the sun fuels our energy. Even how we relate to space - through stillness or presence - shapes our inner balance. The more we live in tune with nature, the more balanced, vibrant and whole we become.

Nature is not separate from us; it is who we are. By embracing its elements, we restore our innate balance and return to the wholeness that is our natural state of being.

The Role of Natural Therapies: Healing Through the Elements

Understanding the connection between the five elements and our well-being lays the foundation for healing through **Natural Therapies**. These therapies harness the power of nature, using earth, water, fire, air and ether to restore balance and activate the body's self-healing mechanisms. Just as the elements shape life itself, they also form the basis of therapeutic practices like hydrotherapy, mud therapy, sun therapy, breath work, fasting and meditation. By working in harmony with nature rather than against it, these methods repair and rejuvenate the body at the deepest level, allowing true healing to unfold.

Mud Therapy: Embracing Earth's Healing Touch:

A full mud bath, or earth wrap, is a common treatment in Naturopathy hospitals. A fine paste of purified mud is applied over the entire body, including the scalp. Initially, many people hesitate. "Mud? On my body?" is a common reaction.

But then the magic begins. As the therapist gently applies the cool, soothing mud, something shifts. At first, there's resistance. Then gradually, relaxation sets in. Tension melts away, and often the most beautiful moment follows…people begin to play. They roll the mud in their hands, shape it and laugh at its texture. The child within, the one who once played in the dirt, built castles and moulded shapes from the soil, comes alive again.

Beyond its physiological benefits - detoxification, better circulation and deep relaxation - mud offers something even more profound. It reconnects us with our innocence, our playful spirit. It's like touching the soil while gardening, with love and care. It reminds us we're not separate from nature; we are part of it.

That's why, among all therapies, mud therapy holds a special place in my heart. It's not just about healing the body; it's about awakening something deep within - our bond with the Earth, with ourselves and with the simple joys we once knew.

Mud: A Gift from the Earth

The more science explores mud therapy, the clearer it becomes that this ancient practice has real, measurable benefits. From detox and pain relief to stress reduction and digestive support, mud's healing potential is vast. Unlike synthetic treatments, mud is simple, natural and deeply rooted in the rhythms of the Earth.

In a world growing increasingly distant from nature, embracing mud therapy revives our connection to natural healing. Whether through a full-body mud bath or a targeted mud pack, the Earth offers us its medicine that is accessible, effective, and deeply grounding.

The Art of Preparing Mud for Healing

Not all mud is suitable for therapy. Healing mud is carefully chosen for purity and potency. It's collected from at least three to four feet below the surface, away from surface pollutants. It's then meticulously filtered to remove stones and debris.

To activate its healing properties, the mud is sun-exposed for a day, enhancing its mineral content. It is then soaked in natural water for at least 12 hours. This final step ensures the mud is hydrated, mineral-rich and ready for therapeutic use, tailored to individual needs.

Mud as Medicine: How It Works

Mud works on many levels, from the surface of the skin to deep within the body. One of its most noted effects is detoxification. With natural adsorptive properties, mud draws out toxins, excess oil and impurities from the skin. As it dries, it pulls debris from the pores, leaving skin clean and revitalised.

Mineral-rich clays like bentonite and Dead Sea mud enhance skin hydration, reduce inflammation and even support wound healing. Research confirms their ability to restore the skin barrier, making them useful for eczema, acne and other conditions.

Beyond skin-deep benefits, mud packs applied to joints or sore muscles reduce inflammation and pain. Peloid therapy – therapeutic mud use – shows positive effects in osteoarthritis and rheumatoid arthritis. The warmth and minerals boost circulation, ease discomfort and improve mobility.

The Nervous System's Response to Mud

Mud therapy also calms the mind. Natural mud contains negatively charged ions, which studies suggest can elevate serotonin, the mood-regulating neurotransmitter. This may explain why contact with mud, soil and natural environments often leaves us feeling refreshed.

Some scientists also highlight the role of beneficial soil bacteria like *Mycobacterium vaccae* in boosting serotonin. This fascinating finding implies that even touching mud could support emotional balance and reduce stress.

Aiding Digestion through Earth's Embrace

A less-known use of mud therapy lies in supporting digestion. In naturopathy, placing a cool mud pack on the abdomen is believed to stimulate digestion and ease bloating or constipation. Cooling the area activates the vagus nerve, vital for gut motility and inflammation control.

Many who use abdominal mud packs regularly report lighter digestion and less discomfort – evidence of the body's positive response to this simple practice.

The Cooling Power of Mud

Mud also serves as a natural coolant. Applied during fever or heat conditions, it helps absorb excess body heat, gradually reducing temperature. This is similar to a cold compress and supports the body's own cooling mechanism.

Naturopathic practitioners have long used mud to soothe fevers and sun-exposed skin, a practice now supported by hydrotherapy and thermoregulation research.

Incorporating Mud Therapy into Daily Life

Mud therapy isn't limited to clinics; it can be part of daily life. Walking barefoot on soil reconnects the body with the Earth, offering physical and mental benefits. Gardening with bare hands builds a healing bond with the land.

Applying a mud pack to the eyes can relieve strain. On the abdomen, it can aid digestion. In inflamed areas, it offers natural relief. These small, intentional acts remind us that healing doesn't always require complexity; often, it lies in our simplest connections with nature.

Hydrotherapy – Water, the Healer

When I was a lecturer teaching the basics of Naturopathy I often began my class on Hydrotherapy with a simple question:

"Does anyone believe water can be a medicine? Have you ever used water to heal?"

Most students would sit silent, unsure. But then, addressing a class mostly filled with girls, I'd ask, "What do you do when you have muscle cramps during menstruation?" Almost instantly, someone would reply, "We use a hot water bag."

That answer would trigger a wave of realisations. One by one, they'd recall how they'd used water to heal – hot water for pain, ice for swelling, steam for congestion, warm water for a sore throat or a cold compress for migraines.

It became a moment of awareness. They'd been using water therapeutically all along- without recognising it as medicine. Water is so deeply woven into daily life that we often take its healing benefits for granted. We wake up refreshed by a neutral bath and unwind with a warm one. When someone faints, our instinct is to sprinkle water on their face – it's an unconscious recognition of water's power to revive.

Water works because it profoundly influences the body. It can stimulate or calm the nervous system, expand or constrict blood vessels to influence circulation or reduce inflammation. It's the base of metabolism, carrying nutrients and flushing out toxins. When used with understanding, water becomes a potent tool for detoxification, rejuvenation and healing.

Hydrotherapy is not just about applying water; it's about realising its potential to restore balance. Whether through hot and cold treatments, baths, compresses or hydration, water has always been a healer. It's nature's simplest, most profound remedy, available, effective and often overlooked.

The Healing Power of Hydration: Why Does Drinking Water Matter?

Most people see water as a simple drink, not medicine. Yet Dr Fereydoon Batmanghelidj famously wrote, *"You are not diseased; you are just thirsty."* Hydration isn't a preference; it's essential for survival. Our bodies are 70–90 percent water, and that water drives every physiological function: carrying nutrients, regulating temperature, flushing toxins, lubricating joints and supporting brain performance.

Water's unique power is its ability to dissolve and move substances. Just as sugar dissolves faster in hot water, temperature changes how water behaves inside us. Once inside cells, it binds to proteins, energises mitochondria and even helps shape DNA. A 20 percent drop in cellular water slows metabolism sharply; at 70 percent, metabolism stops entirely (Clegg 2001). In the right amount and pH, water even acts as an antioxidant.

Dehydration of as little as 2 percent weakens endurance, strength, memory and focus. Those foggy, sluggish moments are often thirst signals. Simple self-checks help: pinch the skin on your hand – if it takes over three seconds to rebound, drink. Press a fingernail – if colour is slow to return, you're likely low on fluids. Persistent sock marks around swollen ankles are another clue.

Staying hydrated is simpler than people think. For most healthy adults, aim for about 240 ml (one cup) of water every hour during the first ten waking hours – roughly two litres – before adding extra for exercise or hot weather. Early-day hydration matches kidney filtration, which is most efficient soon after waking. If you're sweating in a gym, sauna or dry climate, add 240–480 ml for every 20–30 minutes of heat exposure. Feeling dryness in your throat means you're already behind; two quick cups (about 500 ml) help you catch up. In very dry conditions, add electrolytes: a pinch of sea salt and a squeeze of lemon improve water absorption and taste.

Even mild dehydration drags down mood, cognition and physical performance, yet it's one of the easiest problems to fix. Drinking water isn't just about quenching thirst; it's about powering every cell. If you adopt one simple, high-impact habit for better health, make it this: drink enough water, consistently and consciously.

Hydrotherapy - The Healing Power of Water

Hydrotherapy, one of the oldest known forms of treatment, utilises water both internally and externally to maintain health and prevent disease. The term comes from the Greek words *Hydro* (water) and *Therapeia* (healing). This form of therapy takes advantage of water's unique properties to provide medical benefits and relaxation.

Water possesses remarkable properties that make it an effective healing agent. It has the ability to retain and transmit heat efficiently, making it a powerful medium for temperature-based treatments. It exists in various forms – liquid, ice or steam – allowing for a wide range of therapeutic applications. The buoyancy of water reduces gravitational pressure on the body, which is particularly beneficial for individuals with muscle weakness or paralysis. Additionally, water applies natural hydrostatic pressure on the body, promoting better circulation and lymphatic drainage. What makes hydrotherapy even more appealing is its accessibility – water is readily available and affordable, making it an effective treatment that can be practiced at home or in clinical settings.

Dr John Harvey Kellogg, a pioneer in hydrotherapy, emphasised that the body's natural healing force is its greatest asset. Hydrotherapy supports this healing ability by utilising water's physical properties to trigger beneficial physiological responses (Kellogg, 1903). When immersed in water, buoyancy reduces joint stress, making movement easier and less painful. Hydrostatic pressure encourages venous and lymphatic circulation, which helps detoxify the body. Water resistance strengthens muscles during movement, making hydrotherapy an excellent choice for rehabilitation. Temperature variations in water therapy stimulate circulation and influence nervous system responses, producing a profound impact on the body's overall function (Becker, 2009).

The effects of hydrotherapy vary based on temperature, duration and method of application. Warm water treatments, typically ranging from 35°C to 40°C, relax muscles, improve blood flow and support detoxification. A warm bath, for instance, soothes the nervous system and reduces stress. On the other hand, cold water immersion, usually between 10°C and 21°C, invigorates the body, stimulates metabolism and enhances alertness. Many people experience an immediate boost in energy and mental clarity after a cold water session (Tipton et al., 2017).

The Power of Cold Exposure in Hydrotherapy

In my classes, I would explain cold treatments as part of Hydrotherapy with a playful analogy: *"Cold applications are like an affair – you feel excited at first, but if it goes on too long it might turn depressing!"* It always got a laugh and helped make the concept memorable. When used wisely, cold applications are among the most powerful anti-ageing and health-promoting practices. They enhance circulation, activate the nervous system and build resilience. But too much or improper use can cause discomfort or harm. Like everything in life, balance matters.

Cold water applications primarily aim to stimulate and invigorate the body. A brief exposure initially causes blood vessels to constrict, but soon triggers dilation, increasing circulation and oxygen delivery to tissues. This boosts metabolism, speeds muscle recovery and sharpens mental alertness (Sramek et al., 2000). However, extended exposure can lead to numbness and slower reflexes, so moderation is key.

Cold exposure, especially through cold showers or ice water immersion up to the neck, has shown multiple health benefits. Studies reveal it can reduce inflammation, boost metabolism and elevate neurotransmitters like dopamine, norepinephrine and epinephrine (Brazaitis et al., 2014; Haghshenas et al., 2021). These chemicals enhance mood, focus and overall well-being throughout the day.

Dr Susanna Soberg and colleagues in Scandinavia found that just 11 minutes of cold water immersion per week, spread across sessions, provides significant health benefits (Soberg et al., 2021). Participants immersed themselves in uncomfortably cold water up to the neck and allowed natural rewarming afterward. This practice increased brown fat around the heart and clavicles, boosting metabolism and cold tolerance. Their findings also showed noticeable fat loss, especially in the abdominal area.

A compelling study titled *"Impact of Cold Exposure on Life Satisfaction and Physical Composition of Soldiers"* involved 49 participants aged 19 to 30, divided into two groups, one receiving deliberate cold exposure, the other serving as a control. The experimental group underwent one weekly cold immersion (3°C for two minutes) and five cold showers per week (10°C for 30 seconds). Participants warmed up naturally post-exposure. Results showed improved sexual satisfaction, better anxiety regulation and a 5.5 percent drop in abdominal fat after eight weeks, especially in men (Heinonen et al., 2020).

Targeted cold exposure to the upper back and neck during showers is especially effective due to the brown fat concentration in these areas. This type of fat is metabolically active and supports thermogenesis, helping generate heat and reduce white fat (Cypess et al., 2009).

Hot water therapy, in contrast, offers soothing and calming effects. Heat improves circulation and nerve activity, easing pain and muscle tension. Brief hot water exposure promotes relaxation and supports detoxification, but staying in too long may cause fatigue and weaken muscles (Wilcock et al., 2006). Heat therapy is ideal for easing chronic pain, enhancing immune function by increasing white blood cell flow and helping the body conserve energy by briefly lowering metabolism.

Basic Hydrotherapy Treatments

Among the various hydrotherapy treatments, some of the most commonly used are the hip bath, spinal bath and steam bath. The hip bath involves immersing the lower abdomen and hips in water, stimulating circulation and helping in detoxification. It is especially beneficial for digestive disorders, menstrual discomfort and pelvic congestion. The spinal bath, where the patient lies on their back with water covering the spine, is excellent for calming the nervous system, reducing stress and alleviating back pain. Steam baths, available in different forms such as steam rooms and herbal steam therapy, promote deep detoxification by opening the pores, improving circulation and enhancing metabolic function (Mero et al., 2015).

Three Basic Rules of Hydrotherapy Application

The effectiveness of hydrotherapy follows three fundamental principles.

The shorter the application, the more profound the effect - brief but intense exposure to hot or cold water can create a stronger physiological response than prolonged exposure.

- The smaller the area of application, the better the effect - targeting specific areas such as the spine or abdomen can be more effective than full-body treatments.
- Lastly, the greater the temperature difference, the stronger the impact - alternating between hot and cold temperatures enhances circulation and stimulates the body's healing response.
- Understanding these rules allows for precise and effective hydrotherapy treatments tailored to individual needs.

The Sun: Protector and Giver of Life

Since the beginning of time, the Sun has been revered as the ultimate source of life. Ancient civilisations across the globe saw the Sun not just as a celestial body, but as a powerful force that sustains, heals and protects. One of the most profound examples of this reverence is found in the Indian epic *Ramayana*, where the warrior-prince Lord Rama receives a sacred hymn – the *Aditya Hridayam* – from the sage Agastya.

Before Rama's crucial battle with the mighty Ravana, powerful demon king and ruler of Lanka, Sage Agastya shares this powerful *mantra* dedicated to the Sun (Surya). It's more than a prayer; it's a declaration of the Sun's role as the eternal witness, remover of obstacles and source of boundless energy. Chanting it is said to awaken Surya's strength, wisdom and healing power, key qualities needed to overcome challenges.

But is this just mythology, or is there truth behind these beliefs? Modern science confirms that sunlight is indeed a life force. The Sun regulates our circadian rhythms and hormone production, and drives photosynthesis – the foundation of the food chain. Natural light exposure influences mood, metabolism and immunity, while lack of it has been tied to depression, weakened defences and chronic disease.

When we compare the *Aditya Hridayam*'s essence with scientific studies on sunlight's impact, the alignment is striking. Just as the *mantra* sees the Sun as a healer and protector, research shows that sunlight promotes vitamin D production, strengthens bones, improves cardiovascular function and has antimicrobial effects. Infrared and near-infrared rays have been shown to reduce inflammation and support cellular repair, affirming ancient views of the Sun as a healing force.

The wisdom of our ancestors as recorded in sacred texts and holistic practices echoes modern findings. In Naturopathy and Helio (Sun) Therapy, the Sun is more than an external entity; it's a vital element of our well-being. Mindful morning exposure, light-based therapies and reconnecting with nature help us align with life's natural rhythms.

As we explore the Sun's healing power, let's remember that its light lives both outside and within us. Just as it dispels darkness, it energises body, mind and spirit, guiding us toward vitality and inner balance.

The Fire Element as a Healing Agent in Naturopathy

The fire element - symbolised by the Sun and the spectrum of light - holds a vital place in Naturopathy as a potent healing force. Light, as an expression of this element, has long been used to regulate biological rhythms, influence physiological processes and restore balance.

Sunlight is electromagnetic energy that interacts with living systems at multiple levels. Its wavelengths penetrate tissues to varying depths, triggering significant physiological effects that promote healing. Once sunlight reaches the body it's absorbed through two primary pathways - photoreceptors in the eyes and melanocytes in the skin - initiating a cascade of biological responses.

Photoreceptors in the Eyes

The human eye contains rods and cones, photoreceptors that absorb light and send signals to the brain. Blue light, especially in the evening, suppresses melatonin, disrupting sleep, while red light encourages melatonin release, supporting restful sleep. Light exposure helps regulate sleep cycles, mood and cognitive clarity.

Melanocytes in the Skin

Skin cells called melanocytes absorb ultraviolet (UV) light, especially UVB, which is essential for synthesising vitamin D. This vitamin supports calcium absorption, immune function and metabolic health. As an endocrine organ, the skin translates sunlight into hormonal changes, affecting reproductive health, mood and more.

Once light enters the body, all cells respond, directly or indirectly. Red and near-infrared light, for example, reaches deeper tissues, influencing mitochondria. This process, called photobiomodulation, boosts ATP production, reduces inflammation and speeds tissue repair. UVB exposure activates p53, a vital protein for cell repair, and can trigger the release of beta-endorphins, natural pain relievers.

Soaking in the Sunshine – The Truth about Vitamin D and Sunlight

From childhood we've often heard that sunlight is good for us. "Go play outside!" or "Get some sun!" were common phrases. And they weren't wrong. Sunlight truly is nature's medicine, especially when it comes to vitamin D. But here's the surprise: Despite abundant sunlight, 70- 90 percent of Indians are vitamin D deficient. Globally, it's not much better - about 40–50 percent of the world's population has inadequate vitamin D levels.

This isn't just a number; it's a red flag. Vitamin D deficiency is quietly linked to a wide range of health problems, from lifestyle diseases like diabetes and thyroid dysfunction to reduced immunity and mood disorders.

At my clinic, when people come to me in the early stages of lifestyle-related conditions, one of the first things I recommend is checking their vitamin D levels. And more often than not their levels are low, even when they claim to be getting sunlight regularly.

The question is: Why is this happening?

Understanding the Missing Link: Vitamin D and Sunlight

The answer lies in a simple gap – a lack of awareness about how vitamin D is made and what kind of sun exposure is actually needed to produce it.

Vitamin D isn't just a nutrient; it acts more like a hormone in the body. Your skin makes it when exposed to the sun, specifically to UVB rays. It plays a vital role in building strong bones, supporting your immune system, lifting your mood and even protecting against disease.

Here's how it works: When UVB rays hit your skin, a natural substance called 7-dehydrocholesterol (think of it as a sunlight-sensitive chemical) gets converted into vitamin D3. This form is then sent to your liver and kidneys, where it's transformed into its active version: calcitriol. That's the version your body actually uses.

Though we often associate vitamin D with bone health, it is involved in much more. It helps your body absorb calcium, supports immune defence, regulates mood and mental clarity, and even plays a role in preventing chronic diseases.

During the COVID-19 pandemic, researchers began noticing a pattern - low vitamin D levels were linked to worse outcomes. Studies showed that over 80 percent of hospitalised COVID-19 patients were deficient. Other research indicated that people with sufficient vitamin D had lower chances of needing intensive care or dying from the virus.

The Art of Getting Vitamin D from Sunlight

Now, here's the key part – not all sunlight is equal. Many people believe that early morning sunlight is ideal for vitamin D. But the truth is, you need UVB rays, and they are strongest between 10 am and 2 pm. That's right – the midday sun, which many avoid, is actually your best window for vitamin D synthesis.

Just 10 to 30 minutes of sun exposure daily on the face, arms or legs is usually enough. The important part is that the skin must be directly exposed without sunscreen, glass or thick clothing blocking the rays.

But for many, this is easier said than done. Cultural practices, modesty, urban clothing, working indoors and air pollution make proper sun exposure difficult. In addition, sunscreen, while excellent for preventing sunburn, blocks UVB rays, the very rays we need to produce vitamin D.

And if you have darker skin, there's an added challenge. Melanin - the pigment that gives skin its colour - acts like a natural sunscreen. That means you may need longer exposure to produce the same amount of vitamin D as someone with lighter skin. But the more you're exposed, the more your skin darkens, which further reduces vitamin D production. It becomes a bit of a cycle. That's why finding the right balance is so important.

To add to this, unlike many other nutrients, vitamin D is hard to get from food alone. Only a few foods like fatty fish, egg yolks and fortified products offer decent amounts. Even a healthy, balanced diet may fall short. That's why sunlight remains the most reliable and natural source for most people.

What Can You Do?

It's simple, really. Start by stepping into the sunlight, mindfully and regularly. Let your skin absorb the rays it needs. Don't overdo it, and don't try to tan yourself. Just a few minutes every day, especially around midday, can do wonders.

If you live in a region with limited sunlight, work indoors most of the time or wear full-body clothing, it might be wise to get your vitamin D levels tested. If they're low, you may need to supplement, at least for a while.

Remember, **supplements are just that - supplements**. They aren't a replacement for nature, but when it comes to vitamin D, they may be necessary to bring your levels to the optimal range.

Sun-Based Treatments in Naturopathy

Naturopathy has long regarded the sun as a vital healing force, using solar energy through sun-based therapies to promote detoxification, circulation and regeneration. These include sunbaths, banana leaf baths, chromotherapy and infrared radiation therapy, each offering unique benefits. Heliotherapy, or controlled sun exposure, improves circulation, boosts immunity and enhances skin health. Brief, mindful sunbathing stimulates vitamin D production, activates the endocrine system and promotes detoxification through natural perspiration. It's particularly helpful in managing fatigue, arthritis and respiratory conditions.

Banana leaf baths are a traditional treatment where the body is wrapped in banana leaves and exposed to sunlight. This induces sweating, aiding toxin release while the leaves' enzymes nourish the skin. It's especially useful for muscle pain, joint stiffness and skin disorders. At our centre, we call this *Atapa Madhusnana,* a refined practice that begins with a massage using honey and coconut milk, followed by sun exposure in banana leaves. This nourishes the skin and enhances detoxification. Unlike saunas that rely on external heat, *Atapa Madhusnana* activates the body's own thermoregulation, making the process more natural and in tune with physiology. This system, vital for maintaining core temperature, is often weakened by indoor living and air conditioning. Restoring it promotes resilience, energy and overall wellness.

Chromotherapy, or colour therapy, uses the full spectrum of sunlight to affect both body and mind. Each colour carries a unique vibration with targeted effects. Modern research supports this – blue light reduces inflammation and is used to treat acne and certain infections due to its antibacterial and calming effects. Red light, especially low-level red light therapy, improves circulation, accelerates wound healing and boosts collagen production, essential for skin and tissue health. It's also studied for easing arthritis symptoms and enhancing muscle recovery.

Infrared radiation therapy deepens the benefits of light healing. Infrared rays, particularly in the near- and far-infrared range, penetrate deeply into tissues, far beyond the reach of visible light. This deep warmth dilates blood vessels, improves circulation, reduces stiffness and supports detoxification. It eases pain and inflammation gently and effectively. Beyond warmth, infrared light also enhances mitochondrial activity - the cell's energy centres - supporting cellular repair and vitality. This is why it's gaining popularity in physiotherapy, sports medicine and chronic fatigue treatment.

In many naturopathic centres, infrared therapy is paired with sunbathing and traditional oil massages, creating a layered healing experience. The combination of solar warmth and therapeutic oils calms the nervous system, improves lymphatic flow and enhances detoxification. These treatments go beyond symptom relief; they aim to restore the body's inner rhythm and self-healing capacity, often disrupted by modern indoor-centric lifestyles. Sunlight in its many forms remains one of nature's most powerful medicines; when used with care, it becomes a transformative tool for healing and renewal.

The Air Element – The Breath and the Bath

No one needs to be told why we should breathe. It's one of those things that just happens - if you're breathing, you're alive. But here's the catch: While everyone breathes, not everyone breathes correctly, and that's where most of us go wrong.

There's a saying: If you want to understand the importance of something, take it away for a while. But with breathing, we never get the chance to experience its absence - not for long, at least. Since we don't get to pause and reflect on how much we need it, we rarely think about how we're actually doing it.

Breathing keeps us alive by delivering oxygen to our cells, particularly to the brain, which requires a constant supply to function. It also helps remove carbon dioxide, a waste product of metabolism. We all know this much about breathing. However, the way we breathe directly impacts our physical health, mental state and even emotions.

The Unique Power of Breathing

Breathing is special because it sits at the crossroads of the conscious and subconscious mind. Unlike your heartbeat or digestion which happen automatically, you can take control of your breath whenever you want. This ability provides a powerful tool to regulate our body and mind, if we learn to use it properly.

Why Learn to Breathe Correctly?

You can survive without food for weeks and without water for days, but without breathing? Just a few minutes. Does this mean oxygen is more important than food and water? Not exactly. All three are essential. However, while food and water can be stored, oxygen cannot. The body needs a continuous supply at every moment of life.

Yet, oxygen is a double-edged sword. While it sustains life, too much of it - or the wrong kind of exposure - can be harmful. When we breathe, oxygen enters our bloodstream and is delivered to our cells, where it's used to produce energy. In this process, tiny by-products called *free radicals* are created. These are unstable molecules that can damage cells, proteins and DNA if they're not kept in check. Over time, this process - called oxidation or oxidative stress - contributes to ageing, inflammation and various diseases, from cancer to heart disease and accelerated ageing, similar to how a sliced apple turns brown or iron rusts. Proper breathing isn't just about getting more oxygen, but about delivering it efficiently and ensuring that the body uses it optimally.

How to Breathe Correctly

Have you ever wondered if the way you breathe affects your health and well-being? To analyse and understand this, the two major factors to consider are whether you are breathing through your nose or your mouth, and whether you are breathing slow and deep or fast and shallow.

Are you breathing through your nose or your mouth?

Pause for a moment and observe your breathing. Is it nasal or mouth breathing? Is it deep or shallow? This simple observation can reveal a lot, almost like reading your future health.

If you are unsure, try this simple test using the yogic Kechari Mudra:

1. Sit in a relaxed position and take a few slow nasal breaths.
2. Gently roll your tongue backward so that the back of your tongue touches the upper part of your mouth.
3. Maintain this position while continuing to breathe through your nose for about three minutes.

If you can comfortably breathe through your nose without switching to mouth breathing or feeling suffocated, it indicates efficient nasal breathing. If you struggle, it may suggest partial nasal blockage or a tendency to rely on mouth breathing.

Nose vs Mouth: The Two Pathways of Breath

There are only two ways to bring air into the body: through the nose or the mouth. Regardless of the entry point, the air travels down to the lungs, which function like expandable bags, allowing air exchange.

However, the lungs themselves have no muscles to move air in and out. Instead, two key muscle groups control your breath:

1. **The Diaphragm** – A thin muscle located below the lungs. When you inhale, the diaphragm contracts and moves downward, creating more space for the lungs to expand.
2. **The Intercostal Muscles** – These muscles between your ribs contract during inhalation, allowing your rib cage to move outward, further expanding lung capacity.

Proper breathing isn't just about inhaling and exhaling; it's about using these muscles efficiently to maximise oxygen intake and support overall health.

Nose Breathing vs Mouth Breathing: Why It Matters

Breathing through your nose creates more resistance compared to mouth breathing. While this may seem like extra effort, it actually enhances oxygen absorption and overall lung function. Studies suggest that nasal breathing promotes the production of nitric oxide, a gas that relaxes and widens blood vessels, improving circulation and oxygen delivery throughout the body (Lundberg et al., 1996). This ensures better oxygenation of vital organs, including the brain and muscles.

When we breathe through the nose, the air is filtered, humidified and warmed before reaching the lungs. This process enhances oxygenation and overall health. In contrast, mouth breathing bypasses these natural filters, leading to increased dehydration, reduced oxygen absorption and even changes in facial structure. Chronic mouth breathing has been linked to altered jaw alignment, cognitive function issues and a higher risk of sleep disturbances (Becking et al., 2017; Galeotti et al., 2011).

Nasal breathing also plays a crucial role in brain function. When you inhale through your nose, it activates the olfactory system, which detects chemicals in the air and stimulates brain regions involved in learning and memory such as the hippocampus (Zelano et al., 2016). Research published in the *Journal of Neuroscience* found that nasal breathing enhances cognitive function, including reaction time and emotional processing (Zelano et al., 2016).

In contrast, mouth breathing disrupts oxygen supply to the prefrontal cortex, the part of the brain responsible for focus, decision-making and emotional control. This can lead to brain fog, difficulty concentrating and even increased stress or anxiety (Sutcuoglu et al., 2020). Over time, poor oxygenation to this area can impact cognitive function and emotional balance.

Another major downside of mouth breathing is that it causes the body to lose 40 percent more water compared to nasal breathing (Nunn & Anderson, 1983). This can lead to dehydration, especially during sleep, causing frequent urination and disrupting sleep quality. Studies have also linked chronic mouth breathing to increased airway resistance and a higher likelihood of sleep disturbances (Becking et al., 2017).

Beyond health effects, how you breathe can even influence your appearance. Chronic mouth breathing can lead to an elongated jaw, droopy eyelids and a less defined facial structure. Researchers have observed that individuals who predominantly breathe through their mouths may develop features such as a recessed chin and misaligned teeth (Galeotti et al., 2011). However, switching to nasal breathing can lead to improvements in facial features, including better jawline definition and cheekbone structure.

The Takeaway

While nasal breathing requires more effort, the benefits make it well worth the adjustment. It improves oxygen flow, keeps you hydrated, boosts brain function, supports circulation and even enhances facial structure. Making this small change in how you breathe can have a profound impact on your health, sleep and appearance.

Are you breathing slow and deep or fast and shallow?

When I begin my breathing sessions I often start with a simple question: "Does deep breathing increase or decrease the body's oxygen availability?"

The obvious answer most people give is, "It increases oxygen availability." It seems logical – more air should mean more oxygen, right? But let's take a moment to question that.

Imagine a group of us running to the top of a hill. As our muscles demand more oxygen, what happens to our breathing? Do we shift to deep, slow breaths, or start breathing quickly and shallowly? We all know the answer: our breathing speeds up, becoming short and rapid. Now here's the interesting part - if deep breathing were the most effective way to get oxygen, wouldn't our bodies naturally switch to it under stress? But they don't. They use a different strategy.

This raises an important question: If deep breathing is so beneficial, why doesn't the body use it during high oxygen demand? And if fast, shallow breathing takes over during intense activity, is deep breathing less effective than we think?

To understand this, let's compare normal and deep breathing. At rest, most people breathe 12 to 16 times per minute, drawing in about 500 ml of air per breath. That totals around six to eight litres per minute. Now imagine slowing your breath to four to six times per minute, with each breath around 1,000 ml. While each breath takes in more air, the total volume doesn't drastically increase – just slightly more.

So should we still practice deep breathing? Absolutely, but not for the reason most people assume.

The real benefit of deep breathing is improved oxygen utilisation. It's about efficiency. When we slow our breath, we train the body to use oxygen better. Instead of increasing supply, we enhance delivery to our cells.

This is where carbon dioxide – often seen as just a waste product – becomes essential. When oxygen enters the bloodstream, it binds to haemoglobin in red blood cells. But oxygen doesn't release into the tissues on its own. It needs a signal – and that signal is carbon dioxide.

Carbon dioxide or CO_2 changes the shape of the haemoglobin molecule, prompting it to release oxygen. Without enough CO_2, haemoglobin holds onto oxygen too tightly. This is known as the **Bohr Effect**, and it shows that good breathing isn't just about how much oxygen we inhale, but how effectively it's released to cells.

When we breathe too fast, especially through the mouth, we blow off too much CO_2. This might feel like more oxygen is entering the body, but it actually reduces how much oxygen reaches our cells. Slower, deeper breathing through the nose helps retain CO_2 at optimal levels, ensuring oxygen is properly delivered where it's needed.

Breathing well isn't just about lung capacity. It's about creating the right internal environment for oxygen to do its job. Deep, controlled breaths aren't about taking in more air; they're about using it smarter. By balancing oxygen and carbon dioxide, we give our cells the energy they need to function at their best. The key isn't more oxygen, it's better oxygen use.

Air Bathing: Harnessing the Healing Power of Fresh Air

An air bath is the practice of exposing the body to fresh air to enhance circulation, improve skin function and promote overall well-being. While it may sound like a simple practice, its effects are deeply rooted in physiology and thermoregulation. Many early naturopaths, including Sebastian Kneipp and Vincent Priessnitz, advocated for air baths as a method to strengthen the body's natural defences. Modern science also supports its benefits.

The Science

The skin plays a minor role in respiration, contributing about 1 percent of total oxygen intake and carbon dioxide elimination (*Hills, 1974*). Though small, this function reflects the skin's metabolic activity and interaction with the environment. During an air bath, the skin is exposed to fresh air, which enhances natural detoxification processes. Sweat and sebaceous glands become more active, promoting the removal of metabolic waste. The skin's pores also open, improving heat dissipation and thermoregulation.

When the skin is exposed to cool air, blood vessels in the superficial layers constrict (vasoconstriction) to reduce heat loss. After a short period, the body adapts by initiating vasodilation, increasing blood flow to warm the skin. This cycle strengthens the capillary network, improves circulation and helps the body become more resilient to temperature changes.

Cold air exposure also stimulates brown adipose tissue (BAT), a type of fat that generates heat through non-shivering thermogenesis. Studies show that regular cold exposure can increase BAT activity, which is associated with better metabolic health and improved insulin sensitivity (*Virtanen et al., 2009*).

The Role of Negative Ions in Fresh Air

One of the most overlooked benefits of fresh air is its abundance of negative ions, especially in natural environments like forests, mountains and near water bodies. Prakriti Shakti, a clinic of Natural Medicine by CGH Earth, where I work, is nestled in the serene hills of the Periyar Reserve Forest in Kerala. Surrounded by abundant natural elements, we often experience strong winds blowing through the forest, creating a refreshing and slightly chilly atmosphere. This sensation is not just invigorating, but fosters a profound sense of well-being. Many of us have felt this same uplifting effect while walking through a dense forest or along the seashore. One key factor behind this refreshing experience is the presence of negative ions in the air.

Negative ions are molecules that gain an extra electron, making them electrically charged. They are naturally generated by the movement of air, water and sunlight. Research suggests that negative ions have several physiological effects on the body. They improve respiratory health by enhancing ciliary activity in the respiratory tract, helping the body filter out pollutants, allergens and pathogens. This process makes breathing easier and can be particularly beneficial for individuals with asthma or allergies (*Harrison, 2004*). Negative ions also improve the oxygen-carrying capacity of red blood cells, leading to better oxygen delivery to tissues and improved cellular function (*Krueger & Reed, 1976*), resulting in increased energy levels and better metabolic efficiency.

Beyond respiration, negative ions have a direct impact on mental well-being. They influence serotonin levels in the brain, helping to reduce stress, improve mood and enhance cognitive function (*Terman & Terman, 2006*). This is why exposure to fresh air, particularly in natural settings, is associated with feelings of relaxation and mental clarity.

The immune system also benefits from negative ions, as they increase white blood cell activity, strengthening the body's defences against infection (*Shevchuk, 2008*). Regular exposure to ion-rich environments can improve immune function and overall resilience. Additionally, negative ions help neutralise indoor air pollutants. In modern indoor environments, air is often laden with volatile organic compounds (VOCs), electromagnetic radiation and excessive carbon dioxide due to poor ventilation. Negative ions bind and neutralise these pollutants, purifying the air and reducing the toxic burden on the body.

Air baths are not merely an old naturopathic tradition, but a scientifically supported practice that enhances circulation, supports thermoregulation, optimises immune function and improves overall well-being. Fresh air, particularly in nature, is rich in **negative ions** that improve respiratory function, boost oxygen absorption and regulate mood. Regular exposure to these natural elements strengthens the body's resilience and contributes significantly to long-term health.

Space as the Foundation of Energy Flow

Space is the most subtle yet profoundly essential element. It is the vast openness within and around us, the container for all existence. Space is present in the stillness between breaths, in the silence of deep thought and in the boundless sky above. It represents pure potential, allowing all other elements to move and interact harmoniously.

Space is intimately connected with energy. In traditional and holistic healing practices, energy is considered the vital force - vitality, *prana*, chi or life force – that sustains the body and mind. The presence of space is necessary for energy to circulate freely. Without space, there is congestion, stagnation and ultimately, disease. In traditional naturopathic philosophy, lowered vitality is seen as the foundation of disease. Healing in Naturopathy is fundamentally about restoring and enhancing vitality rather than just treating symptoms.

Reflexology

Reflexology is a powerful healing method that focuses on applying pressure to specific points on the hands and feet, which correspond to different organs and systems in the body. By stimulating these reflex points, blocked energy is released, allowing the body's natural healing mechanisms to function optimally. Walking on a pebbled reflexology track further enhances this effect, as the varying pressure on nerve endings stimulates corresponding internal organs, improving circulation and pain tolerance over time. This form of therapy is not only beneficial for internal organ function, but also helps build resilience to pain by gradually improving sensory adaptation and nerve response.

Massage Therapy

Massage in Naturopathy is designed to work on the body's soft tissues to stimulate circulation, relax muscles and release stored tension.

Unlike conventional massage, which often focuses on oils and fragrances, naturopathic massage prioritises specific movements and pressure techniques that align with the body's energy pathways. These massages enhance detoxification, facilitate deep relaxation and improve lymphatic drainage, thereby helping restore balance and vitality. Different types of massage, such as deep tissue, lymphatic drainage and rejuvenation massage serve a distinct purpose, but all contribute to the free flow of vital energy within the body.

Acupressure and Acupuncture

Both acupressure and acupuncture are based on the ancient concept of meridians, energy pathways that run throughout the body. These therapies work by stimulating specific points along these meridians to clear blockages and restore balance. Acupressure uses precise, firm pressure applied by hand, whereas acupuncture employs fine needles to activate energy points with greater precision. These techniques not only aid in pain relief and organ function, but also play a significant role in regulating the nervous system, improving sleep and reducing chronic stress. By working on these pathways, acupressure and acupuncture create space for energy to move unobstructed, allowing the body to heal naturally and efficiently.

The Power of Pause

One of the most fundamental yet overlooked therapeutic aspects in Naturopathy is the power of pause, which is a way of using the space element. The modern lifestyle is filled with constant activity, overstimulation and stress, leaving little room for true restoration. Naturopathy intentionally integrates pauses into healing programmes to allow the body and mind to reset and rejuvenate. Practices such as *Upavasa* (fasting) provide a break from sensory attachments, particularly food, allowing the digestive system to rest and detoxify. *Asana* (yogic postures) introduces a pause in movement, promoting flexibility, balance and awareness of bodily sensations. *Pranayama* (breath regulation) creates intentional pauses in breath, which help regulate energy, enhance oxygenation and calm the nervous system. *Dhyana* (meditation) facilitates a pause in thoughts, reducing mental clutter and fostering emotional clarity. *Mauna Vrata* (silent day) is a practice of refraining from speech, allowing individuals to reconnect with their inner self and experience the power of stillness.

By embracing these pauses, the body is given the space it needs to recover and rejuvenate. The intentional act of slowing down, whether through fasting, breath control or silence, helps conserve and redirect energy toward healing. Space, both external and internal, serves as the foundation for health, allowing movement, energy flow and transformation to unfold naturally. When we make room for pause in our lives, we create the necessary conditions for vitality to flourish and for true healing to take place.

★ ★ ★

Naturopathy is about feasting your body with the very essence of nature. The five natural elements - earth, water, fire, air and ether - are not just external forces, but vital energies that communicate with our cells most effectively, guiding the body toward balance and healing. When we align ourselves with these elements, we create an internal harmony that fosters true well-being.

Equally important is the environment we live in. It shapes our health, either nourishing or depleting us. Disease often arises when we disconnect from nature's rhythm, and healing becomes difficult when we remain in the same conditions that led to illness. That is why we say you can never truly heal in the same environment where you became diseased. Change, whether in habits, surroundings or mind-set, is essential for transformation.

Embracing nature's wisdom is not just a practice, but a way of life, one that empowers the body's innate ability to heal, thrive and sustain well-being.

References

1. Chevalier, G., Sinatra, S. T., Oschman, J. L., & Delany, R. M. (2012). Earthing: Health implications of reconnecting the human body to the Earth's surface electrons. *Journal of Environmental and Public Health.*
2. Fioravanti, A., et al. (2011). Mud-bath therapy in knee osteoarthritis: A randomized, controlled study. *Clinical Rheumatology.*
3. Lowry, C. A., et al. (2007). Identification of an immune-responsive mesolimbocortical serotonergic system: Potential role in regulation of emotional behavior. *Neuroscience.*
4. Perez,V., et al. (2013). Airborne negative ions and their effects on human health and behavior. *International Journal of Molecular Sciences.*
5. Proksch, E., et al. (2005). Bathing in a salt-rich Dead Sea solution improves skin barrier function, enhances stratum corneum hydration, and reduces inflammation in atopic dry skin. *International Journal of Dermatology.*
6. Takakura, K., et al. (2015). Vagus nerve stimulation for the treatment of digestive disorders. *World Journal of Gastroenterology.*
7. Clegg, J. S. (2001). Cryptobiosis – a peculiar state of biological organization. *Comparative Biochemistry and Physiology Part B: Biochemistry and Molecular Biology*, 128(4), 613-624.
8. Becker, B. E. (2009). "Aquatic Therapy: Scientific Foundations and Clinical Rehabilitation Applications." PM&R, 1(9), 859-872.
9. Kellogg, J. H. (1903). *Rational Hydrotherapy: A Manual of the Physiological and Therapeutic Effects of Hydriatic Procedures.*
10. Mero, A., et al. (2015). "Effects of steam and sauna bathing on recovery and health." Journal of Human Kinetics, 49(1), 33-41.
11. Sramek, P., et al. (2000). "Human physiological responses to immersion into water of different temperatures." European Journal of Applied Physiology, 81(5), 436-442.
12. Tipton, M. J., et al. (2017). "Cold water immersion: kill or cure?" Experimental Physiology, 102(11), 1335-1355.
13. Wilcock, I. M., et al. (2006). "The effects of water immersion on recovery from exercise." Sports Medicine, 36(9), 747-765.
14. Holick, M. F. (2007). "Vitamin D deficiency." *New England Journal of Medicine*, 357(3), 266-281.

15. Lucas, R. M., & Ponsonby, A. L. (2013). "Ultraviolet radiation and health: friend and foe." *Medical Journal of Australia*, 198(8), 431-433.
16. Juzeniene, A., & Moan, J. (2012). "Beneficial effects of UV radiation other than via vitamin D production." *Dermato-Endocrinology*, 4(2), 109-117.
17. Hamblin, M. R. (2017). "Mechanisms and applications of the anti-inflammatory effects of photobiomodulation." *APL Bioengineering*, 1(1), 011002.
18. Byrne, H. J., & Shand, N. C. (2021). "Red and near-infrared light therapy for human health and wellness: A review." *Photochemistry and Photobiology*, 97(3), 527-549.
19. Becking, B. E., et al. (2017). The impact of obstructed breathing on sleep and craniofacial growth. *European Respiratory Journal.*
20. Galeotti, A., et al. (2011). Mouth breathing: Effect on facial and dental development in children. *European Journal of Paediatric Dentistry.*
21. Lundberg, J. O., et al. (1996). Nasal nitric oxide in man. *Thorax.*
22. Nunn, J. F., & Anderson, K. (1983). Respiratory heat and water exchange. *Physiological Reviews.*
23. Sutcuoglu, T., et al. (2020). The effects of mouth breathing on cognitive function and attention in children. *Journal of Clinical Pediatrics.*
24. Zelano, C., et al. (2016). Nasal respiration entrains human limbic oscillations and modulates cognitive function. *Journal of Neuroscience.*

CHAPTER 9

The Conductor

Rhythm: What Turns Noise into Music!

As we enter a new phase in our journey toward health and healing, we have explored various concepts and practices on how to do the right things. However, these right actions become truly effective only when performed at the right time – that is what rhythm is all about.

Nothing in our body happens randomly. Every function is interconnected, forming part of a grand, controlled plan. Just as the rhythm of sound creates music, the rhythm of life creates health. Our body follows natural cycles, known as biological rhythms, which regulate everything from sleep and digestion to hormone production and energy levels. These rhythms are influenced by nature, time and our daily habits. Understanding and aligning with them can significantly enhance our well-being.

The Circadian Rhythm: The Cycle of Day and Night

One of the most well-known rhythms is the circadian rhythm, which follows a 24-hour cycle. This internal clock governs our sleep-wake cycle, metabolism, hormone release, digestion and even immune function. Our body is naturally programmed to wake up with sunlight and wind down as darkness sets in. Disrupting this cycle by staying up late, exposing ourselves to artificial light at night or eating at irregular times can lead to fatigue, poor digestion and hormonal imbalances. Living in alignment with the circadian rhythm, such as sleeping early and getting morning sunlight, supports overall health.

There are people who call themselves 'night owls'. Funny, isn't it? No matter how much you call yourself an owl, you are still human!

And as a human, your body demands a natural cycle of wakefulness and sleep based on its biological rhythms.

The circadian rhythm is the body's internal clock that governs the 24-hour cycle of physiological and psychological functions. It is primarily regulated by light and darkness and is deeply connected to hormone regulation, body temperature, digestion, immune function and mental well-being.

Morning sunlight exposure is equally essential, as the sun acts as the master regulator of the body's internal clock. Viewing light through windows is not as effective, because glass reduces light intensity significantly. Direct exposure to sunlight is necessary to properly set the circadian rhythm. When daylight enters your eyes, it signals to a specific centre in the brain, known as the suprachiasmatic nucleus (SCN), which acts as the master clock. This signal prompts the release of cortisol, the hormone responsible for wakefulness and energy. Cortisol levels peak in the morning, ensuring alertness and focus, while exposure to natural sunlight during the day strengthens this rhythm and prepares the body for better sleep at night.

As the sun sets and darkness takes over, the SCN triggers the release of melatonin, the sleep hormone. Melatonin prepares the body for rest by reducing alertness, lowering body temperature and promoting relaxation. However, exposure to artificial light, especially blue light from screens, confuses the brain and delays melatonin production, leading to difficulty falling asleep and poor sleep quality.

A well-regulated circadian rhythm supports overall health, but when it is disrupted the body suffers. Daylight plays a vital role in energy levels, as sunlight exposure boosts serotonin, a neurotransmitter that enhances mood, focus and motivation. Without sufficient sunlight, people often feel fatigued, irritable and unmotivated. Melatonin is equally important in regulating body functions. When its production is disturbed, sleep patterns become erratic, leading to insomnia, stress and metabolic imbalances.

The consequences of poor sleep extend beyond tiredness. Inflammatory conditions such as arthritis worsen due to increased production of pro-inflammatory cytokines. The body's ability to repair tissues occurs primarily during deep sleep, so inadequate rest leads to pain, stiffness and an overall decline in physical health. Mental and emotional well-being are also deeply tied to circadian balance. Disruptions increase the risk of anxiety and depression, while chronic sleep deprivation impairs cognitive function, memory and emotional stability.

Maintaining a healthy circadian rhythm requires a regular sleep and wake schedule. Sleeping in complete darkness is crucial, as studies show that even one night of sleeping in a moderately lit environment increases heart rate, decreases heart rate variability and raises next-morning insulin resistance. These findings indicate that even while asleep, exposure to dim light disrupts the nervous system and cardiometabolic functions, emphasising the importance of darkness for quality sleep.

Additionally, following a natural rhythm supports overall well-being, including sexual health. Melatonin, the hormone that helps us wind down and sleep, naturally rises when it gets dark. While it's essential for good rest, melatonin also influences the part of the brain that controls our reproductive hormones. At night, when melatonin is higher, it temporarily slows down the signals that trigger the production of hormones like testosterone and oestrogen. This is completely normal; it's the body's way of prioritising rest and recovery during night time.

But if melatonin levels stay high during the day – like when we don't get enough sunlight or are exposed to too much artificial light at night – it can throw off the balance. Over time, this may affect sex hormone levels and lower libido. So it's not that melatonin itself reduces sex drive, but when our natural rhythm is off, it can have ripple effects on things like mood, energy and sexual health.

You are not an owl, and we can't follow the rhythm of owls or any other birds or animals. We are human, and our body thrives when we honour its natural demands. Respect your circadian rhythm, and it will reward you with energy, vitality and longevity.

Ultradian Rhythms: The Short Cycles That Keep Us Going

While the circadian rhythm sets the stage for our daily wake-sleep cycle, our body also follows ultradian rhythms – shorter cycles that occur multiple times a day. You might not realise it, but your focus and energy naturally rise and fall in 90-minute alertness-rest cycles. This is why working for long hours without breaks leaves you feeling mentally foggy and drained. Your brain needs moments of rest between these cycles to stay sharp.

Digestion too operates in ultradian digestive cycles. Eating at random times, when you are not feeling hungry, can throw your system off balance, but when you follow a natural rhythm – having meals at regular intervals – your body can digest and absorb nutrients more efficiently.

Your heart rhythm is another ultradian cycle. Your heart naturally adjusts its rate based on your activity, stress levels and emotional state. A well-regulated heart rhythm, known as heart rate variability (HRV), reflects a body that is resilient and adaptable. When you're calm and at ease, your heart beats in a more harmonious way, promoting overall well-being.

Even your respiratory rhythm follows a predictable pattern. Every inhale and exhale influences oxygen levels, brain function and your nervous system's balance. When you breathe deeply and steadily – especially through your nose – you feel more centred and focussed. But shallow, erratic breathing can trigger stress and fatigue. That's why breath work practices like *pranayama* help restore balance, calming the mind and nourishing the body with oxygen.

Infradian Rhythms: The Longer Cycles That Shape Us

Beyond the daily and hourly rhythms, our bodies also follow longer cycles known as infradian rhythms. One of the most well-known is the menstrual cycle, which spans roughly a month and influences everything from energy levels to mood and metabolism. These natural hormonal shifts are part of a woman's biological rhythm, shaping how she feels and functions across the weeks.

But women aren't the only ones affected by infradian rhythms. Our bodies also respond to the changing seasons. Seasonal metabolic changes impact our metabolism, sleep patterns and even immune function. You may notice that in winter your body craves heartier foods and more rest, while in summer you feel lighter and more energetic. This is the body's way of adapting to the natural world.

The Subtle Rhythms of Nature

Beyond these major cycles, there are more subtle rhythms that influence our well-being, such as lunar rhythms and tidal rhythms. Some traditions believe the moon's phases impact emotions, sleep and even bodily fluids. Meanwhile, tidal rhythms, which mirror ocean tides, may influence fluid movement and detoxification processes within the body.

Each of these rhythms – whether short, long or tied to nature's elements – plays a role in our health and vitality. By tuning into these cycles, we can make choices that support our body's natural harmony. Instead of fighting fatigue, we can honour our need for rest. Rather than forcing a rigid eating schedule, we can follow our body's cues. Life itself is a rhythm, and when we move in sync with it, we thrive.

CHAPTER 10
The Destination

Thank you for walking this path of health and healing with me. This journey has never been about extremes or restrictions; it has been about embracing balance, growth and the beauty of continuous transformation. Healing is not a single moment of change; it is a gentle unfolding, a journey of self-discovery that happens every day.

In my roadshows, I often say:

Healing programs are like taking a bath – they cleanse what has already gathered, but life continues, and so we bathe again the next day. Similarly, the journey of health and healing is a daily, ever-evolving process.

This path may bring challenges, but these are not roadblocks – they are stepping stones. Every challenge is an opportunity to grow stronger, wiser and more in tune with yourself. Without these moments, we would never truly understand our own strength.

Healing is about releasing what no longer serves you, letting go of anything that weighs you down and stepping into the fullness of who you are meant to be. It is about shifting from uncertainty to awareness, from hesitation to action, from waiting to embracing the present moment. We all dream of a healthier, happier life, but dreams come to life when we create a plan and take steps to make it real.

This journey is also about discovery – unlearning old patterns that no longer support you and relearning habits that nourish your body, mind and soul. It is an invitation to take charge of your own well-being. You are your greatest healer.

Healers and doctors are here to walk beside you, to encourage, support and guide you toward a life of vitality. But the real transformation happens within you, when you tune into your body's wisdom and listen to the intelligence that already resides within you.

Let these reminders inspire you:

The enemy of healing is fear.
The thief of joy is comparison.
The termite of relationships are assumptions.
The saboteur of peace is expectations.
Anger sets fire to the self.

Be mindful of these truths, and let them uplift you.

As we reflect on this journey...
Healing is not about rushing to the finish line. It is all about moving in the right direction, not about speed. Like cooking a nourishing meal, healing takes patience – rushing the process may give the illusion of progress, but true transformation happens when we allow ourselves the time to heal fully and deeply.

Let us conclude with the **Shanti Mantra** from the *Brihadaranyaka Upanishad*, a universal prayer of compassion, harmony and well-being resonating with the essence of holistic healing and inner balance:

सर्वे भवन्तु सुखिनः
सर्वे सन्तु निरामयाः ।
सर्वे भद्राणि पश्यन्तुः
मा कश्चित् दुःखभाग भवेत् ॥
ॐ शांतिः शांतिः शांतिः॥

(Sarve Bhavantu Sukhinah
Sarve Santu Niramayah
Sarve Bhadrani Pashyantu
Ma Kashchid Dukhabhag Bhavet
Om Shantiḥ Shantiḥ Shantiḥ)

May all beings experience happiness and well-being. May everyone be free from illness, suffering and disease. May all witness and experience what is auspicious, noble and uplifting in life. May no one, anywhere, ever suffer or endure pain.

Om Shanti, Shanti, Shanti – may there be peace and harmony in the universe, in the environment and within ourselves.

About the Author

Dr Cijith Sreedhar, BNYS, MSc (Yoga), Certified NLP Practitioner, has over 17 years of experience guiding people toward holistic health and natural well-being. As Chief Medical Officer at Prakriti Shakti – Clinic of Natural Medicine by CGH Earth, Kerala, a NABH-accredited Naturopathy & Yoga hospital, he combines medical expertise with a passion for empowering individuals. He has represented Naturopathy & Yoga internationally and contributes to national policy and accreditation initiatives through the Ministry of AYUSH. He currently serves as National Coordinator of the Indian Naturopathy & Yoga Graduates Medical Association (INYGMA).

A sought-after speaker, educator and researcher, Dr Cijith has delivered his signature talk, *Awaken the Healer Within,* across India, the Middle East and Europe. His work has been published in journals such as the *Journal of Lifestyle Medicine and Frontiers in Pain Research*, and featured in the *Deccan Chronicle*, *Vogue* and *The Week*. By blending modern science with ancient wisdom, he inspires people to tap into their body's innate healing power – cultivating strength, balance and vitality.

You can contact Dr Sreedhar at drcijith@gmail.com or on +91 85900 17785.